Healthy Eating in the 21st Century

Your Simple Guide to Eating Healthy in the Modern World

by Devin Burke, CHHC, CPT

MEDICAL DISCLAIMER

This book is for reference and informational purposes only and is no way intended as medical counseling or medical advice. The information contained herein should not be used to treat, diagnose or prevent a disease or medical condition without the advice of a competent medical professional. The author, writer, editors, and graphic designer shall have neither liability nor responsibility to any person or entity with respect to any damage or injury alleged to be caused directly or indirectly by the information contained in this book. You should consult your doctor before starting any nutrition program.

How to get the most out of this book:

1. Set an intention. To prepare for the journey ahead, take some time to clarify your health goals and reasons for choosing to read this book.

2. Read each chapter in chronological order.

3. Review the key concepts found at the end of each chapter.

4. Most important, implement the action items and use the chapter supplemental materials.

5. Visit **www.healthyeating21.com**, enter your name and email to receive book updates and the latest healthy eating in the 21st century information.

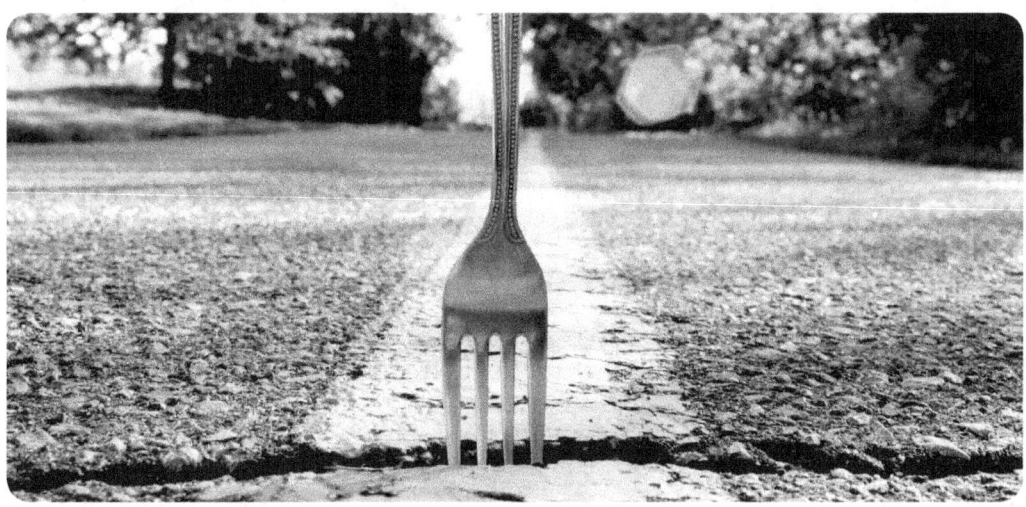

About the Author

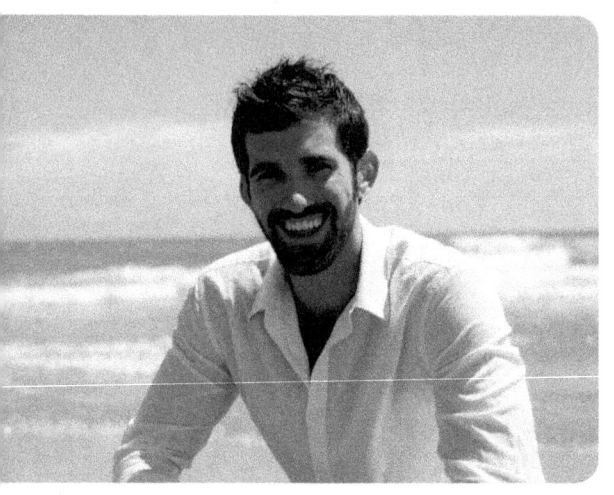

Devin Burke is a passionate wellness educator, health and fitness coach, and the founder of Empowerment Wellness Solutions, a healthy lifestyle coaching business based in South Florida. After graduating from Florida Atlantic University, with a major in Exercise Science and Health Promotion, he furthered his education at the Institute for Integrative Nutrition. He has studied over 100 dietary theories, practical lifestyle management techniques, and innovative coaching methods with some of the world's top health and wellness experts. Through his education and passion to help others, Devin has transformed and inspired many lives. Devin's life mission is to inspire and educate as many people as he can to experience optimal health.

Devin is a Certified Holistic Health Coach, a Certified Personal Trainer by the American College of Sports Medicine, and a Therapeutic Exercise Technician. Through his education, he has extensive knowledge in holistic nutrition, health coaching, exercise science, and preventive health. He specializes in lifestyle coaching, as well as functional strength training. He believes that true wellness is achieved through finding balance in mind, body and spirit, and he is committed to sharing his message with the world. His goal in creating this book is to provide a simple, yet practical guide to eating healthy in the 21st century.

DevinBurke.com

Table of Contents

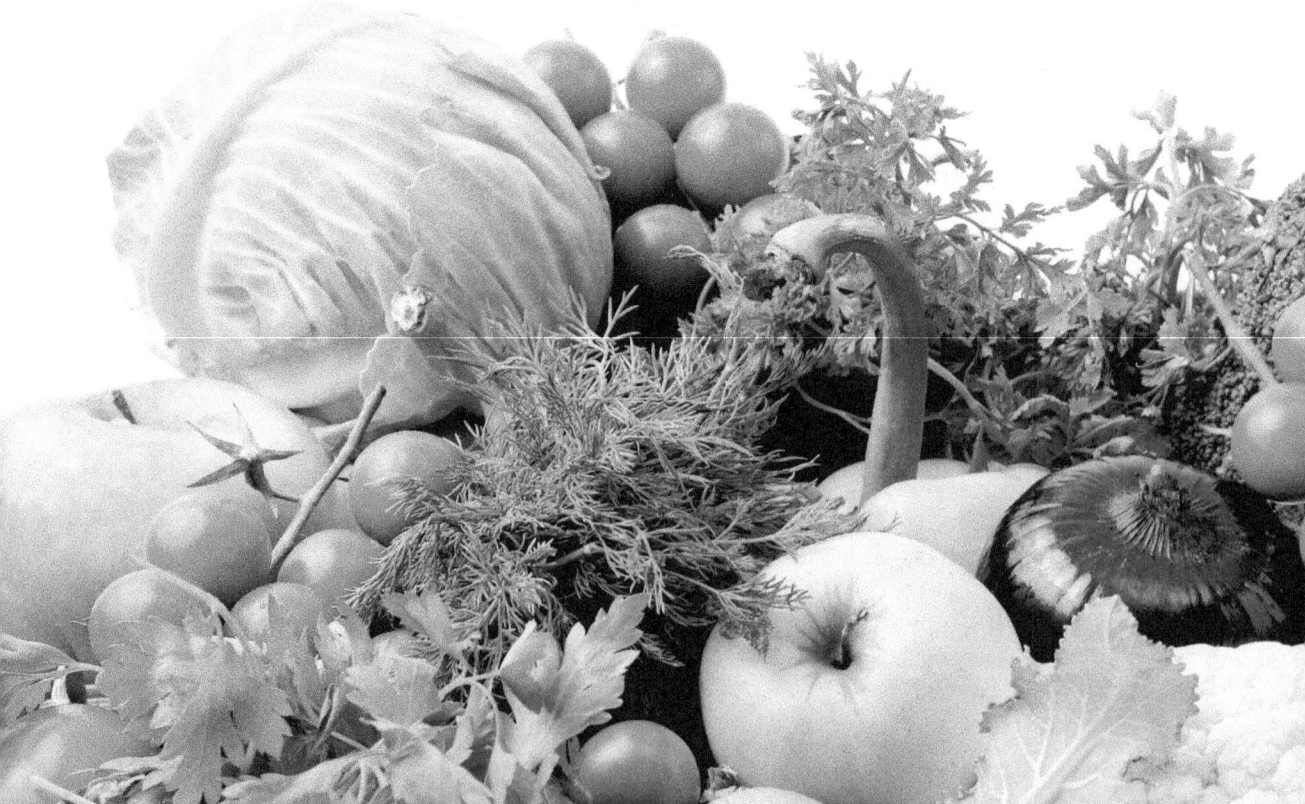

Welcome to Healthy Eating in the 21st Century

Congratulations!

You have just made an extraordinary commitment to your health and wellness. This book was designed with your health and lifestyle in mind. Throughout the book, I will guide and educate you on the fundamentals of eating healthy in the 21st century.

I believe knowledge is power. When you are informed and educated you have the power to take action. Right now, fully commit to taking immediate and massive action to change your life by not only educating yourself, but by really implementing the strategies and solutions you'll find throughout this book.

In this book, I will uncover the scary truth about our food production methods and how to avoid harmful foods. You will be educated on what real food is and how to start including more real food into your diet. Together, we will discover strategies and techniques for meal planning and preparation, food shopping and label identification, so that you can immediately apply what you are learning to greatly improve your energy, mental clarity and overall health. You'll also find amazing information for eating healthy on-the-go, such as when traveling or attending social events. Then, we'll cover some amazing, healthy recipes and meal options to keep your taste buds inspired.

It's time to start giving yourself the fuel your body and mind needs to drive you towards looking and feeling your absolute best.

Please read and sign the following agreement as a commitment to yourself to fully get the most out of this book.

I am committed to my own personal health and wellness.
With this commitment I give my word to...

1. Be open to new foods and concepts
2. Make changes that will greatly improve my health and life
3. Follow the action items at the end of each lesson
4. Eat more nutrient dense nourishing foods according to the guidance of this book

_____   _____
Please sign here.   Date

1

WHAT NOT TO EAT
Dangers and Misinformation in Our Current Food System

We all eat every day, but somehow, most people are really quite confused about what to eat. Despite all the nutritional research, diet books and theories, how is it that most Americans are still baffled about what to eat to achieve a long and healthy life?

Well for starters, nutrition is the only field where people can scientifically prove opposing theories and still be right. That being said, we've come a long way in understanding how the food we eat affects our health.

But, due to food politics, the food industry in this country resembles a battle field of politics and greed. Public nutrition policy is commanded by the political process, which is orchestrated by large food corporations, all to maximize their profits with little regard for our health.

The truth is that the majority of food we are eating is not really food at all, but rather engineered processed food that puts dollars in the food corporations' pockets and leaves the rest of us overweight, diabetic or worse. Sadly, about 70% of the calories Americans are eating today come from processed artificial foods.

These foods are making us fat, sick and tired. Between misleading food marketing, untruthful labels and a food industry with a focus on profits and not health, we are experiencing a global health epidemic. But there is hope on the horizon because you have the power to not only educate yourself on what foods will truly nourish your mind and body, but to vote with your dollar. As we continue into the 21st century, let's commit to changing the health of the world by first changing ourselves. **Small choices lead to big changes**. Let's make a big change together by discovering how to eat healthy in the 21st century.

Let's get started.

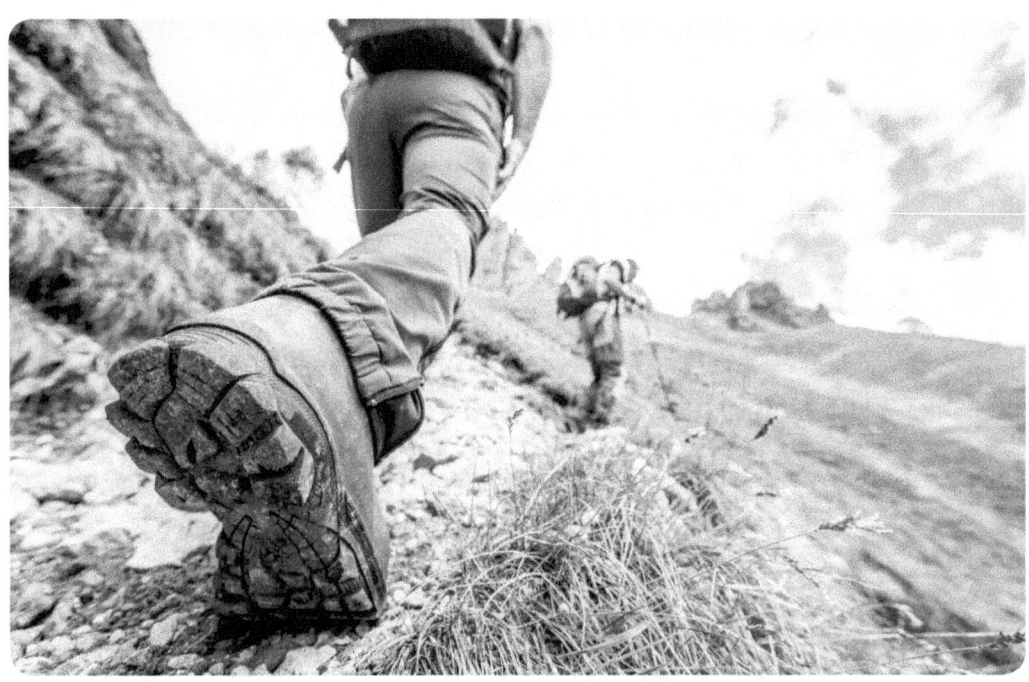

In this chapter, I hope to permanently change the way you view conventional and processed foods by not only providing you with real information on why eating these types of foods negatively impacts your health, but also by bringing awareness to the current dangers of our food production methods.

Originally, all food was grown and prepared without pesticides, herbicides, chemical fertilizers, genetic engineering, hormones, antibiotics or the preservation process of irradiation. Foods were unrefined, whole and minimally processed...the way nature intended them to be.

Today, it's a very different story. Today, the vast majority of our food is grown conventionally, which means it is sprayed with pesticides, herbicides, and all types of other dangerous chemicals. It is grown using the process of genetic modification, preserved with the process of irradiation and injected with antibiotics and hormones. Conventionally grown and processed food is far from what nature intended us to eat. So what does all this mean and why should you care?

Have you ever heard the saying, "you are what you eat?" Well, it's true! We literally are what we eat. Our food goes into our stomachs, it's digested and absorbed into our blood. Our blood is what creates our cells, tissues, organs, even our thoughts. So we not only feel and look differently based on what we eat, we actually think differently. For this reason, it's extremely important to know how the food you eat was grown and where it came from.

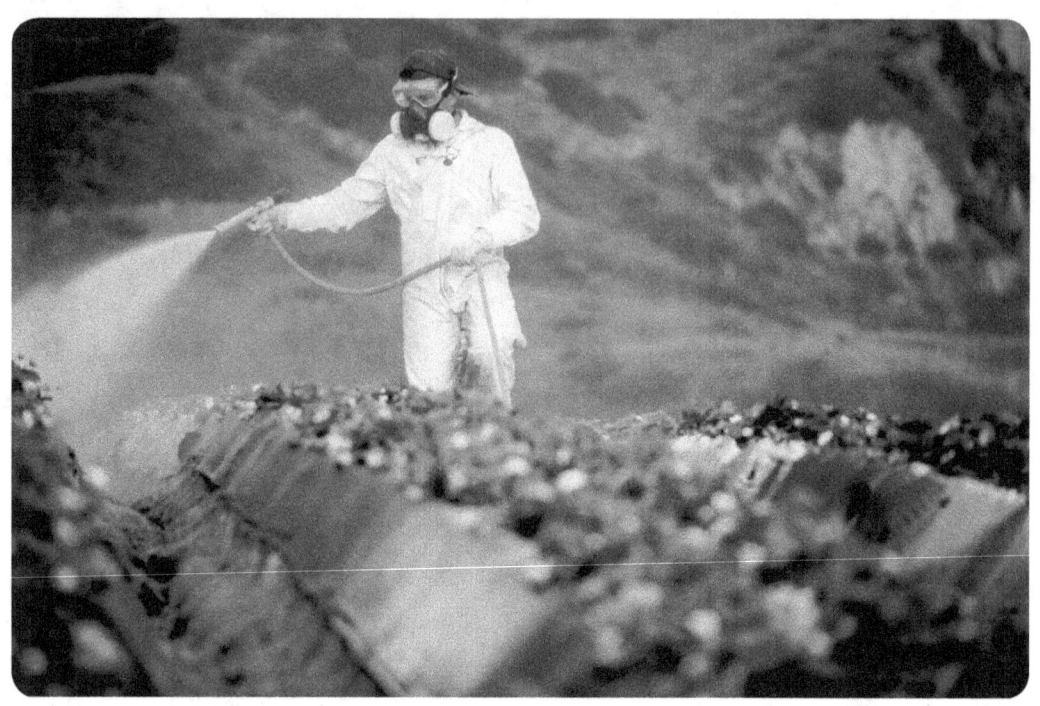

Pesticides

Pesticides are poisons designed to kill living organisms and thus are harmful to humans. Many pesticides that are still being used today were approved long before research linked these chemicals to diseases such as cancer. Today, there are hundreds of pesticides approved for use in the United States that present different health risks. While some are linked with cancer, others are known to cause birth defects, harm the nervous system and disrupt the delicate hormone (endocrine system). Our body's endocrine system is highly sensitive. We use hormones to coordinate just about everything that takes place in the body—from cell growth, to appetite and metabolism. A scary reality is that every year **more than two billion pounds** of pesticides are added to our food supply. [1] That's about 10 pounds per person per year! Now, more energy is actually used to produce synthetic fertilizers than to till, cultivate and harvest all the crops in the U.S. and three billion tons of topsoil erodes from crop lands in the U.S. each year, due to conventional farming practices. [2] Conventional farming practices also ignore the health of the soil, which is where food gets its nutrients.

When pesticides are sprayed on our food, trace chemical residues of these pesticides after consumption lodge and accumulate in our body tissue, which weakens our immune system and leaves us susceptible to disease. Another scary reality is that research shows that children are up to **4 times** more sensitive to exposure to cancer-causing pesticides in foods than adults and 1:3 adults will be diagnosed with cancer and that number is steadily increasing. [3] By consuming food that has been exposed to these dangerous farming chemicals, you are putting your health and the environment at risk. Avoid eating conventional food when and where possible.

---

[1] Earth Island Journal. "The Spraying of America." www.Earthisland.org N.P., Nov 2014 Web.

[2] EZIAHP. "Top 10 Reasons to Buy and Eat Organic Foods." www.ESIAHP.com, Sept. 2012 Web.

[3] Natural Resource Defense Council. "Our Children at Risk." www.nrdc.org, Nov 1997 Web.

More Scary Facts about Pesticides

The U.S. Department of Agriculture strictly prohibits mixing different types of pesticides for disposal, due to the well-known process of the individual chemicals combining into new highly toxic chemical compounds. 62% of food products tested contained a measurable mixture of residues of at least three different pesticides.[1]

1. Conventional blueberries tested positive for 42 different pesticide residues.

2. 64 different pesticides have been found on conventionally grown grapes.

3. 78 different pesticides were found on conventionally grown lettuce samples.

According to the Environmental Protection Agency's (EPA's) "Guidelines for Carcinogen Risk Assessment," **children receive 50% of their lifetime cancer risks in the first two years of life.** According to the EPA and the National Academy of Sciences, standard chemicals are up to **4-10 times more toxic** to **children** than to adults, depending on body weight. This is due to the fact that children take in more toxic chemicals relative to body weight than adults and have developing organ systems that are more vulnerable and less able to detoxify toxic chemicals. [1]

---

[1] Healthy Holistic Living. "Just the Facts Please." Top Facts about Organic Foods. www.healthy-holistic-living.com N.P., 11 Oct 2014 Web.

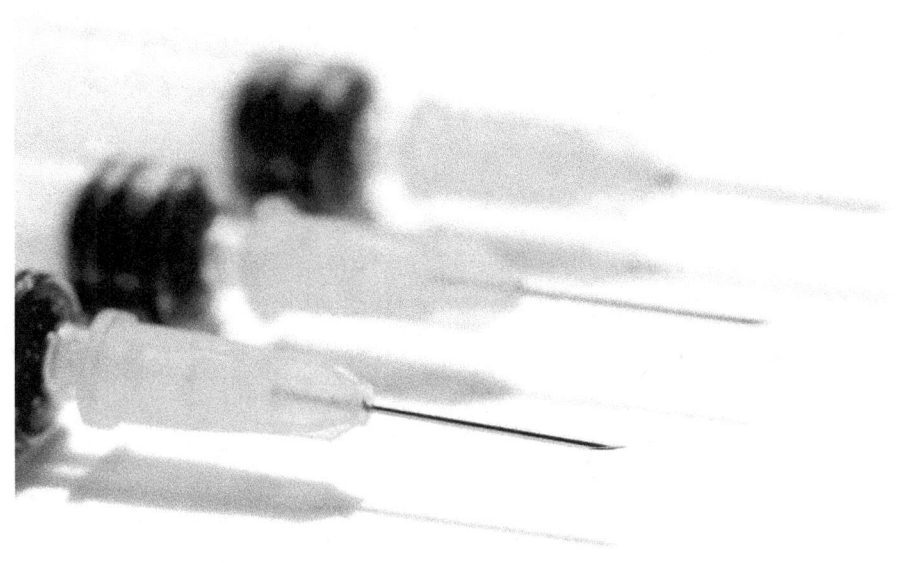

Hormones and Antibiotics

Due to factory farming, almost all conventionally grown animals today have been injected with antibiotics and growth hormones. This is to increase production and, therefore, the profits of the companies using these methods. Unfortunately, when we consume these animals, we're exposing our bodies to those same hormones and antibiotics. Scientists now have clearly shown that these hormones can increase the risk of disrupted development and cancer in humans. The use of antibiotics has encouraged a new evolution of new strains of antibiotic-resistant bacteria in our food supply. [1] This is extremely detrimental to not only our environment but also to our health. Avoid eating conventionally farmed animals when and where possible to limit your exposure to harmful hormones and antibiotics.

More Scary Facts about the Use of Hormones and Antibiotics in Factory Farming:

1. A typical supermarket chicken today contains more than twice the fat and about 1/3 less protein than forty years ago due to the unnatural diet and hormones used in the farming process.

2. Nine out of ten U.S. calves are treated with hormonal growth promoters. [2]

3. The FDA has approved five hormone implant growth promoters for cattle. Three of them – estradiol, progesterone and testosterone – are naturally occurring hormones that are identical to those found in humans.

4. One of the five hormones used in U.S. cattle, Zeranol, caused a significant spurt in tumor growth; even at levels thirty times lower than levels the FDA maintains are safe. [2]

5. The European Union (EU) has refused to import U.S. beef from animals treated with hormones. [2]

---

[1] Today's Dietitian. "Antibiotics in Animal Agriculture." Experts Weigh in on a Meaty Issue. www.Todaysdietian.com N.P., June 2010 Web.
[2] Mother Earth News. "What You Need to Know About the Beef Industry." Are Hormone Implants Safe? www.motherearthnews.com N.P., 11 Oct 2014 Web.

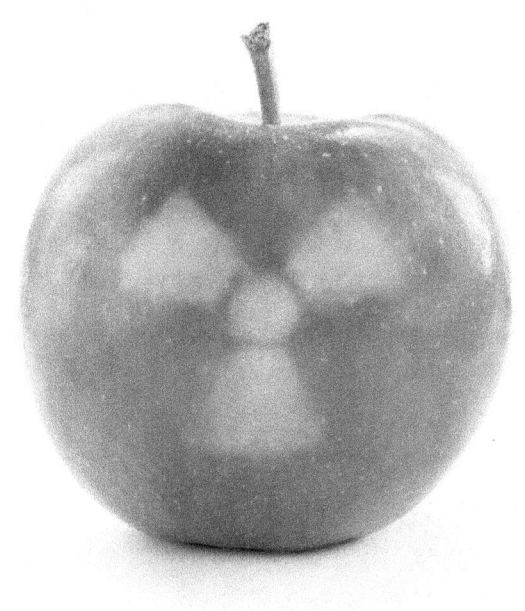

Irradiation

Irradiation is another questionable method used in the preservation of today's conventional foods. These foods are treated with ionizing radiation from Cobalt 60, Cesium 137, X-rays or high energy electron beams from machine sources. This is far from natural. Other terms commonly used to identify ionizing irradiation are "cold pasteurization" and "irradiation pasteurization." Ionizing radiation reduces the number of disease-causing organisms in foods by disrupting their molecular structure and killing potentially harmful bacteria and parasites. However, when food is irradiated, some nutrients are destroyed and untested compounds, referred to as URPs (unique radiolytic products) are created. [1]

Four Reasons Why the Process of Irradiation is Harmful:

1. Irradiation damages the quality of food. Irradiation damages food by breaking up molecules and creating free radicals. The free radicals kill some bacteria, but they also bounce around in the food, damage vitamins and enzymes, and combine with existing chemicals (like pesticides) in the food to form new chemicals. [2]

2. Scientists have not studied the long-term effects of these new chemicals in our diet. Therefore, we cannot assume they are safe for human health. The longest human feeding study was fifteen weeks. No one knows the long-term effects of a life-long diet that includes foods which will be frequently irradiated. [2] It's important to note that irradiated foods can lose up to 5%-80% of many essential vitamins like (A, C, E, K and B complex). The amount of vitamin loss depends on the dose of irradiation and the length of storage time.[2]

3. Irradiation damages the natural digestive enzymes found in raw foods. This means the body has to work harder to digest them. Studies on animals fed irradiated foods have shown increased tumors, reproductive failures and kidney damage. Some possible causes are: irradiation-induced vitamin deficiencies, the inactivity of enzymes in the food, DNA damage and toxic unique radiolytic products or URPs in the food. [2]

4. Irradiated foods can have longer shelf lives than non-irradiated foods, which means they can be shipped further while appearing 'fresh.' Food grown by giant farms far away may last longer than non-irradiated, locally grown food, even if it is inferior in nutrition and taste. Thus, irradiation encourages centralization and hurts small farmers. [2]

[1] Whole Foods. "Irradiation (US and Canada)." Whole Foods Market and Irradiation. www.wholefoodsmarket.com N.P., 10 Oct 2014 Web.
[2] Organic Consumers. "What's Wrong with Food Irradiation." www.organicconsumers.org N.P., Feb 2001 Web.

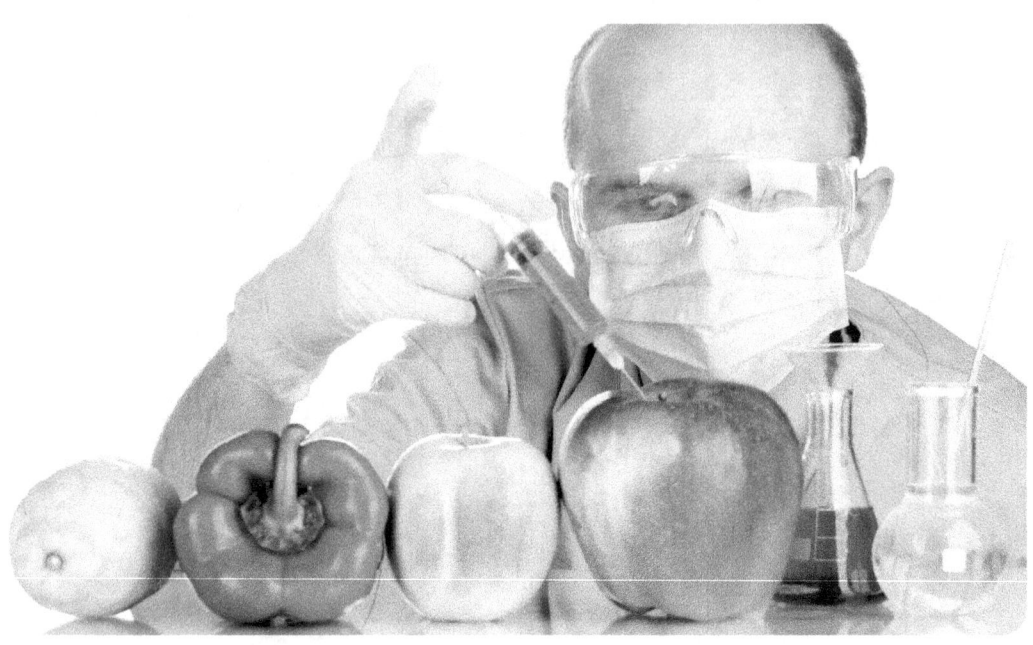

Genetically Modified Organisms (GMOs)

A genetically modified organism or GMO is a plant or animal that has been genetically altered by scientists to express different characteristic traits. In the case of agriculture, it's to improve a crop's ability to grow in certain conditions. [1] For example, the most common use of genetic engineering in agriculture is to create pesticide-resistant plants, which then allows farmers to use more farming chemicals on their crops without killing them. There is a growing body of evidence that now connects GMOs with health problems and environmental damage. Interestingly, most developed nations do not consider GMOs to be safe. In fact, in more than 60 countries around the world, including Australia, Japan and all of the 28 countries in the European Union, there are significant restrictions and bans on the production and sale of GMOs. Avoid eating GMOs when and where possible to avoid putting your health at risk.

More Reasons to Avoid GMOs:

1. Long term studies haven't been done on their impact on the human body. GMOs have only been in our diet since mid 90's. [2]

2. Genetic modification forces genes to express different traits, which can release allergens normally not expressed in the non-GMO species.

3. GMO seeds require pesticides, resulting in the use of more cancer causing pesticides sprayed on foods. [1]

4. GMOs are connected with increased risk of cancer, reproductive issues and autism. [2]

5. GMOs pollute our clean air, water and soil. [1]

6. GMOs can destroy natural plant varieties in the wild through cross-pollination.

---

[1] Non GMO Project. "What is GMO?" Agricultural Crops that Have a Risk of Being GMO. www.Nongmoproject.org N.P., Oct 2014 Web.
[2] Naturally Savvy. "What's so bad about GMOs?" Top Ten Reasons to Avoid Them. www.Naturallysavvy.com N.P., Oct 2014 Web.

PROCESSED ARTIFICIAL FOOD

As a nation, we are overfed but undernourished. We are literally starving from a nutrition basis. This is because 70% of Americans' diets consist of processed artificial foods. [1] The scary reality: Not getting enough essential nutrients in a way our bodies can recognize, absorb and assimilate leads to nutritional starvation and disease.

Processed artificial foods are the aftermath of man's failed attempt to mimic real food and have been concocted in a lab and even worse, usually engineered to be addictive! The sad truth is that food companies now actually engineer addictions into the foods they create and there is no law banning companies from doing this. **Their goal is to not make healthy food products, but rather ones that we'll continually buy, have a long shelf life, and will make them a profit.**

Processed artificial food products may look like real food, but they are far from what nature intended us to eat. They are loaded with refined sugars, trans-fats and all types of other artificial chemicals to make them look and taste similar to real food at the expense of our health. Processed artificial foods or what I refer to as man-made "food-like" products, actually can trick our bodies into thinking they are getting specific nutrients, but they are not nourishing our bodies at the cellular level. This leads to disease. **Avoid eating artificial processed foods when and where possible!**

---

[1] Market Place. "Processed Foods Make up 70 percent of the U.S Diet." www.marketplace.org March 2013 Web.

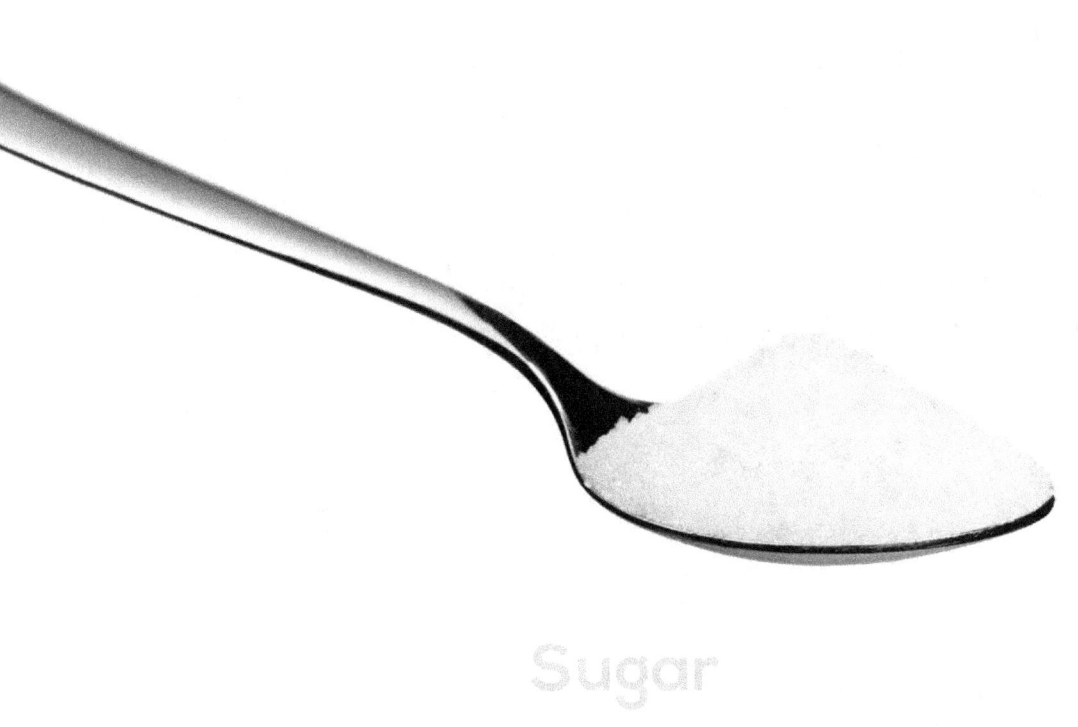

Sugar

It's scary that Americans consume about 150 pounds of sugar per year and 80 pounds of those 150 pounds are in the form of high fructose corn syrup. [1] That's about ½ pound a day per person. High fructose corn syrup is the unhealthiest kind of sugar because it's absorbed more rapidly than regular sugar and doesn't stimulate ghrelin or leptin production, the "hunger" and "full" signaling hormones, which leads to overconsumption of food and disease. Research has now linked excessive amounts of sugar to cancer, diabetes and heart disease.

Unfortunately, sugar is found in almost everything, even "healthy" products today; and when sugar isn't used or burned, it's stored as fat in the body. Sugar also causes inflammation in the body, and inflammation is at the root of almost all chronic diseases today. But even worse than refined sugar and high fructose corn syrup is chemical artificial sweeteners such as Splenda (sucralose), Sweet & Low (saccharin), Equal and NutraSweet (aspartame). These sugar substitutes have been created in a lab and recently linked to a long list of related negative side effects, such as headaches, nausea, anxiety, depression, dementia, skin rashes and cancer. Start reading labels of the products you're buying...even the "healthy" ones. To maintain optimal health, avoid processed refined sugars and sugar substitutes.

Sugars to Avoid: refined sugars (sucrose), high fructose corn syrup, artificial sugars (Splenda, Sweet & Low, Equal and NutraSweet)

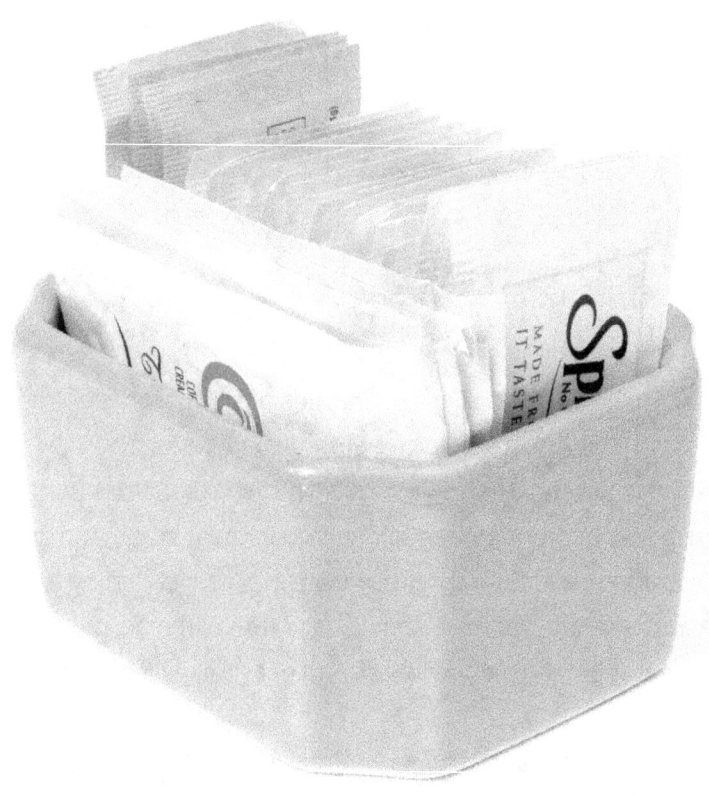

1] Medicine Net. "The Hidden Ingredient That Can Sabotage Your Diet" Do You Know How Much Sugar You're Eating? www.Medicinenet.com N.P., Sept. 2014 Web

The worst kind of fat is trans-fat or trans-fatty acid, also known as partially-hydrogenated oil. Most trans-fats are created industrially by adding hydrogen bonds to liquid oils to make a more shelf-stable product. However, some trans-fats occur naturally in beef, lamb, butterfat and dairy. Trans-fats raise LDL (bad cholesterol) and lower HDL (good cholesterol). When a fat molecule is partially-hydrogenated, the body doesn't recognize it and the fat is carried around in the blood which leads to plaque buildup in the arteries which leads to heart disease.

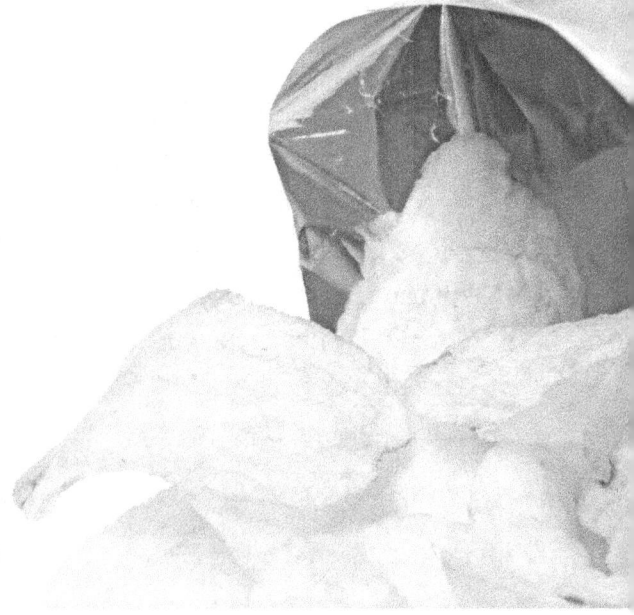

When reading labels, your eyes may be trained to search for "trans-fat," but there are some loopholes food manufacturers are allowed in order to sneak trans-fat into their products. Although a product may say '0g trans-fat,' this may not be true. Only foods and supplements with 0.5g of trans-fat and greater are required to be listed on the food label. Next time you browse a label, search the ingredient list for the term 'partially hydrogenated' and pass it up if you find it on the label. [1]

Trans-fat may be found in margarine, processed foods, candy, chips, soda, flaky pastries and some peanut butters.

---

[1] "Trans-fat." American Heart Association. N.P., 29 Oct 2010 Web. 17 Feb 2012

As you are aware, quick and portable foods are the norm in today's fast paced society. Unfortunately, most of these foods contain artificial chemical ingredients and additives to preserve their shelf life. These convenience foods or what I call "food-like" products aren't really foods at all. The easiest way to avoid these type of dangerous ingredients is to stay away from packaged foods and eat whole, fresh foods. However, when buying packaged food, just look for any unpronounceable ingredients on the label. This usually is a good indicator that it's artificial. Below is a list of the most detrimental artificial chemical ingredients to look out for.

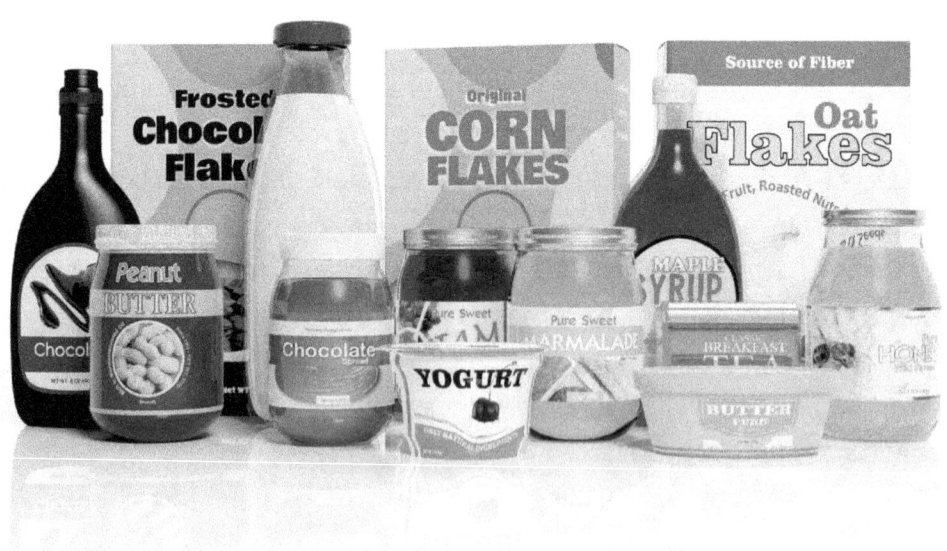

1. **Artificial sweeteners**: related side effects such as headaches, nausea, anxiety, depression, dementia, and skin rashes.

2. **Refined sugars**: High consumption of sugar and the corresponding elevated insulin levels can cause weight gain, bloating, fatigue, arthritis, migraines, lowered immune function, obesity, cavities and cardiovascular disease. [1]

3. **Monosodium glutamate (MSG)**: MSG is a common food additive used to enhance flavor in a variety of foods. Canned vegetables, frozen entrées, fast foods and soups are just a few products that contain MSG. Many people have experienced a variety of side effects ranging from headaches, itchy skin and dizziness to respiratory, digestive, circulatory and coronary issues. [2]

4. **Artificial colors and flavoring**: Food coloring and flavoring is usually a synthetic chemical produced by scientists to color foods and increase a product's visual appeal. Many colorings are derived from coal tar and can contain up to ten parts per million of lead and arsenic and still be generally recognized as safe by the FDA.[2] Artificial colors can cause allergic reactions and increase hyperactivity in children with ADD. [3]

5. **Butylated hydroxyanisole (BHA) and Butylated hydroxyuene (BHT)**: BHA and BHT are two food additives commonly used in the food industry to prevent oils from going rancid. Studies have shown that BHA has caused stomach-focused carcinogens in trials involving mice, hamsters and rats. The U.S. Department of Health and Human Services has deemed BHA "reasonably anticipated to be a human carcinogen." [4]

6. **Sodium nitrate and nitrite**: Sodium nitrate and nitrite are preservatives that are added to processed meat products to enhance red color and flavor. These compounds transform into cancer-causing agents called nitrosamines in the stomach. Noticeable side effects include headaches, nausea, vomiting and dizziness. [4]

7. **Partially hydrogenated oils (trans-fats)**: Partially hydrogenated oils are made by reacting different varieties of oil with hydrogen. When this occurs, the level of polyunsaturated oils (good fat) is reduced and trans-fats are created. These oils are added to products to enhance appearance and prevent spoiling. They are associated with heart disease, breast and colon cancer, atherosclerosis and elevated cholesterol. [5]

---

[1] Kam, Katherine. "The Truth about Sugar." WebMD. N.P., n.d. Web.

[2] Zeratsky, Katherine. "Monosodium Glutamate (MSG): Is it Harmful?" WebMD. N.P., n.d. Web.

[2] Arnell, Neev. "The Dangers of Artificial Food Colors." Natural News. N.P., 25 Mar 2011 Web. 6 Feb 2012.

[3] Franco, Virginia. "Effects of Artificial Colors in Children with ADD." Livestrong. N.P., 25 Mar 2011 Web.

[4] "Food Additives." Center for Science in the Public Interest. N.P., n.d. Web.

[5] Bruen, Jude. "Partially Hydrogenated Oil vs. Hydrogenated Oil." Livestrong. N.P., 29 Nov 2009 Web

GLUTEN

Recently there has been a lot of press around gluten. Gluten is a protein found in several types of grains, including wheat, spelt, rye and barley. It's the glue-like substance that gives bread its elastic properties. Gluten isn't technically harmful to your health unless you have celiac disease, the most severe gluten allergy, or have a gluten sensitivity.

When you have Celiac disease, the immune system attacks gluten and the cells of the digestive tract. It is classified as an autoimmune disease and can lead to nutrient deficiencies, digestive issues, fatigue and an increase risk of many other diseases. It is believed to afflict about 1% of people with over 80% not even knowing they have it. [1]

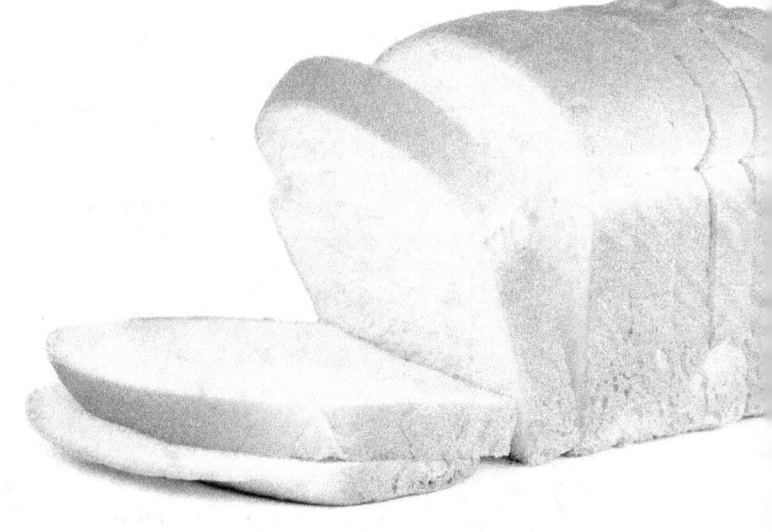

The other type of gluten intolerance is called gluten sensitivity and is much more common. Those who are sensitive to gluten have adverse reactions such as headaches, brain fog, bloating and fatigue. It has been estimated that around 6%- 8% of people have gluten sensitivity. [1]

If you have any of the above symptoms or suspect you may have a sensitivity to gluten, simply eliminate it from your diet for 14 days, then reintroduce it and see how your body responds.

Note: Many processed artificial foods contain gluten. By avoiding these foods, you will lose weight, have more energy and generally feel better. If you're someone who eats a lot of processed foods, avoid all processed foods for 14 days then reintroduce a healthy food item that contains gluten such as whole grain bread and see how your body responses. It may not be the gluten you're sensitive to, but rather something else in the "fake" processed chemical food.

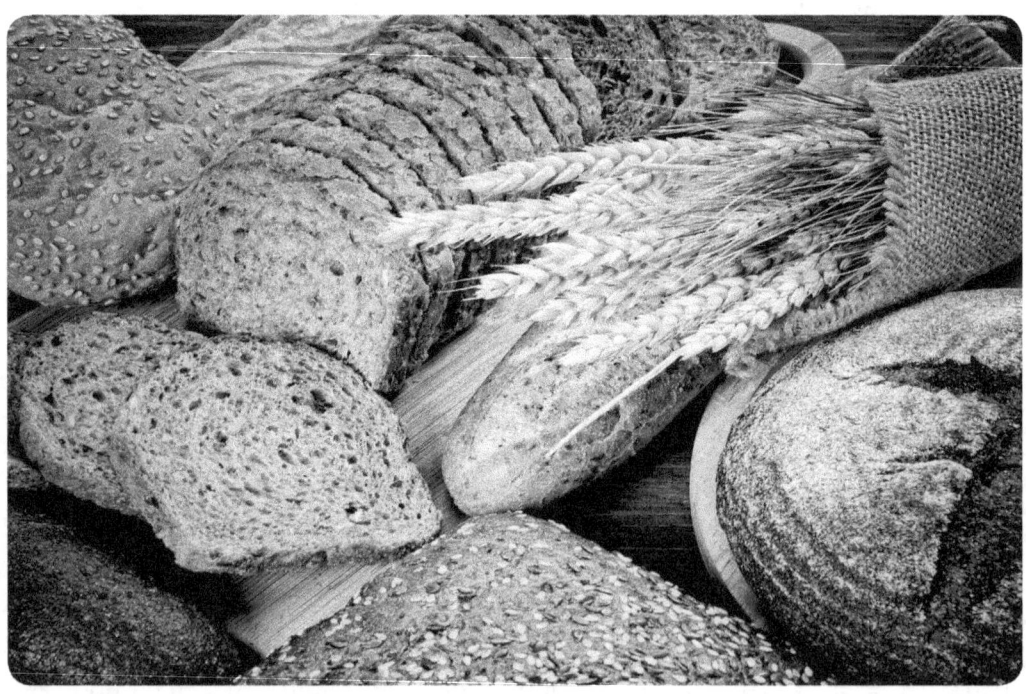

[1] Authority Nutrition. "6 Reasons Why Gluten May be Bad for You." www.authoritynutrition.com, N.P., Nov 2013 Web.

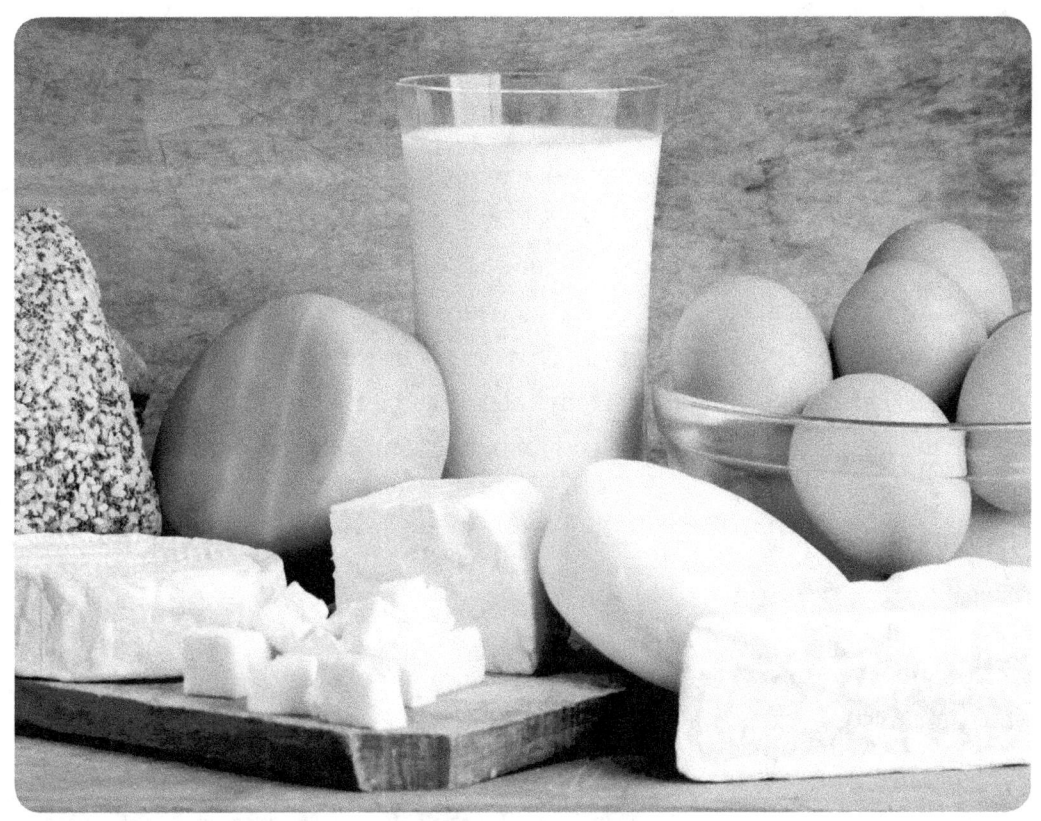

DAIRY

Dairy is another controversial food. Conventional farmed dairy products contain harmful synthetic contaminants like antibiotics, growth hormones and pesticides. Conventionally farmed cows are also fed genetically modified feed and are inhumanely treated to increase production and profits of the companies using these methods.

There are many ethical and environmental implications to how these cows are being raised and treated. Conventional animal agriculture is also a major contributor to global warming and pollution of our water and air. [1]

You may be wondering what about organic dairy products? Well, buying and consuming organic dairy products is definitely a step up from buying conventional dairy products. When you buy organic dairy, you're limiting your exposure to harmful hormones and antibiotics, pesticides and GMO fed cows. However, 30-50 million American adults are lactose intolerant, which means they can't process or break down lactose (milk sugar). Most Americans are not even aware that they are lactose intolerant. Consuming lactose when you're lactose intolerant can cause gas, bloating, diarrhea, and vitamin and mineral deficiencies. Also dairy products are acid forming and can leach minerals out of our bones. [2]

I recommend avoiding dairy products. However, if you find dairy works for your body, make sure you're supporting farms that are producing dairy responsibly by using organic farming methods and treating their cows humanely.

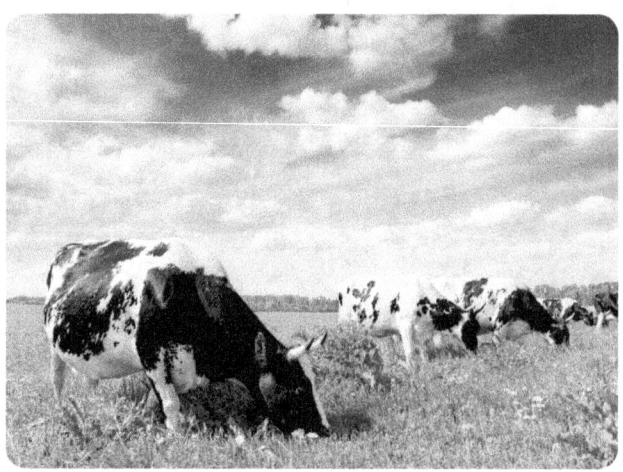

[1] FAO Newsroom. "Livestock, a Major Threat to Environment" www.fao.org N.P., Nov 2006 Web.

[2] Precision Nutrition. "All about Dietary Acids and Bases." www.Precisionnutrition.com N.P., Nov 2014 Web.

HOW FOOD COMPANIES ARE DECEIVING YOU

"People are fed by the food industry which pays no attention to health, and treated by the health industry which pays no attention to food"

- Wendell Berry

Engineered Foods

Food manufacturers are smart. They spend millions of dollars a year to create foods that we will not only want to buy, but will keep us coming back for more. They engineer addictions into their food products. Their goal is to not make healthy food products, but to make foods products that you will continually buy, have a long shelf life, and will make them a profit. We are eating these "food like" products which are causing immune dysfunction. They look and smell like food, but they are far from what nature intended us to eat.

The food manufacturers fund studies stating that their food creations are safe to consume. These results are then presented to the FDA. The FDA then evaluates the studies that the food manufacturers submit. There is often no third party testing for safety or quality.

De-evolution

We are biologically programed to seek calories from fats and sugars. It's a survival mechanism . Our ancestors' biggest challenge was to survive, and in order to do that they needed to find food... food that was high in calories. But the food our ancestors were eating was also high in nutrients.

Today as you now know, our food is depleted of nutrients. However, we are still biologically programmed to put on fat when food is available. The challenge today is that food is always available and it's not good nutritious food, but rather chemical, artificial "fast" food. This has led to the process of de-evolution.

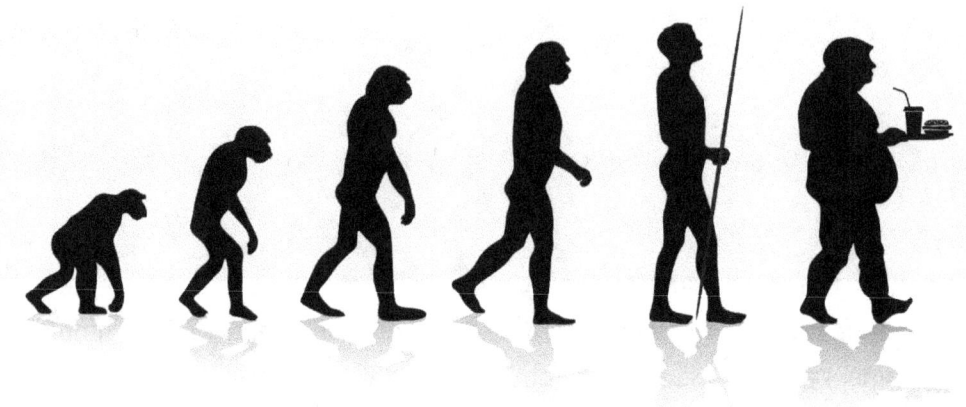

Overfed, but Undernourished

With the majority of people eating foods that are high in calories but low in nutrients, it's no wonder we're experiencing an obesity epidemic and healthcare crisis in America today. Most people are starving from a nutritional basis. This is why our bodies are constantly searching for food, because they want nutrients not calories. Today our calorie sources are coming mainly from unnatural fats and sugars which our bodies are just storing as fat. You can eat 10,000 calories a day, but if you are not getting specific nutrients in a way your body can recognize and assimilate you're starving from a nutritional basis. .As long as you're starving from a nutritional basis, you're going to stay hungry. Our bodies are constantly searching for food because they want nutrients not calories. Think about it, 1,000 years ago you wouldn't find Twinkies hanging from trees. If it doesn't come directly from the ground or a tree, eat it in moderation if at all.

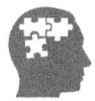

Key Concepts

---

1. Our current food production system is dangerous and not sustainable. Today the vast majority of our food is grown conventionally, which means it is sprayed with pesticides, herbicides and all types of other dangerous chemicals. Conventional farming practices ignore the health of the soil, which is where our food gets its nutrients.

   Unhealthy Soil = Nutrient Depleted Plants = Nutrient Depleted People = Disease.

2. We literally are what we eat. Our food goes into our stomachs, is digested and absorbed into our blood, which then creates our cells, tissues, organs, even our thoughts. We feel and think differently based on what we eat. The better the quality the food, the better the quality the YOU.

3. Processed artificial food products may look and smell like real food, but they are far from what nature intended us to eat. They are loaded with refined sugars, trans-fats and all types of other artificial chemicals to make them look and taste similar to real food at the expense of our health. Avoid all processed artificial foods and food chemicals.

Action Items

✔ Clean out your refrigerator and cabinets of all food-like products. If you find anything that is processed and has a list of ingredients you can't pronounce, it's time to get rid of it.

✔ Review all chapter 1 course materials to get comfortable with controversial ingredients to avoid when food shopping.

✔ Research local farmers markets in your town or city where you can buy organic and local food or a natural grocery store that carries fresh organics. See the supplemental natural food directory resource worksheet guide [pg 60] to assist you in this process.

CHAPTER 1:
SUPPLEMENTAL MATERIALS
Most and Least Contaminated Produce

Many people can't afford to buy all organic all the time. You don't have to buy all organic produce to reduce your risk for chemical contamination. This list from the Environmental Working Group tells you which fruits and vegetables contain the most chemicals and which ones are least contaminated. Use it when shopping to help make the best choices for you and your family – even if you can't buy entirely organic foods.

Most Contaminated Buy Organic!	Least Contaminated
1. Apples	1. Onions
2. Celery	2. Pineapple
3. Strawberries	3. Avocado
4. Peaches	4. Mango
5. Spinach	5. Eggplant
6. Nectarines	6. Kiwi
7. Grapes	7. Watermelon
8. Sweet bell peppers	8. Grapefruit
9. Potatoes	9. Cantaloupe
10. Blueberries	10. Honeydew melon
11. Lettuce	
12. Kale/collard greens	

*If you eat the skin of the produce item, buy it organic when possible!

Source: Environmental Working Group, www.ewg.org

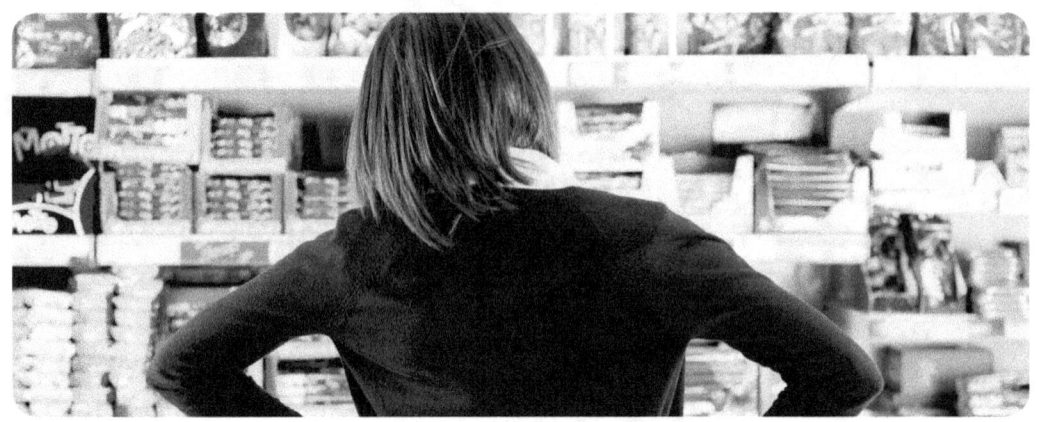

4 Simple Effective Ways to Eat Less Processed Food

1. **Avoid conventional food packaged in boxes, bags and cans.**

   Foods that come in packages are **usually** highly processed. Most are dehydrated, bleached and enriched.

   Note: Some healthy food is packaged in a box, bag and can. See the art of understanding "health" food labels worksheet to learn more (pg 102).

2. **When buying boxed, bagged or canned food, buy food items with 5-10 ingredients or less.**

   Processed foods are loaded with all kinds of unpronounceable food chemicals and ingredients. If you can't pronounce it, you probably shouldn't be eating it.

3. **Shop the perimeter of the grocery store.**

   The perimeter of the grocery store is where you'll find the fresh produce and meat items. The center aisles are usually filled with processed artificial junk food. Beware! Even the "healthy" grocery stores carry a great deal of processed food disguised as health food.

4. **Watch out for "low-fat," "lite," "light," "reduced fat," and "non-fat" food marketing terms**

   These food marketing terms are usually a dead giveaway that the food is highly processed with artificial sweeteners, sugar or both.

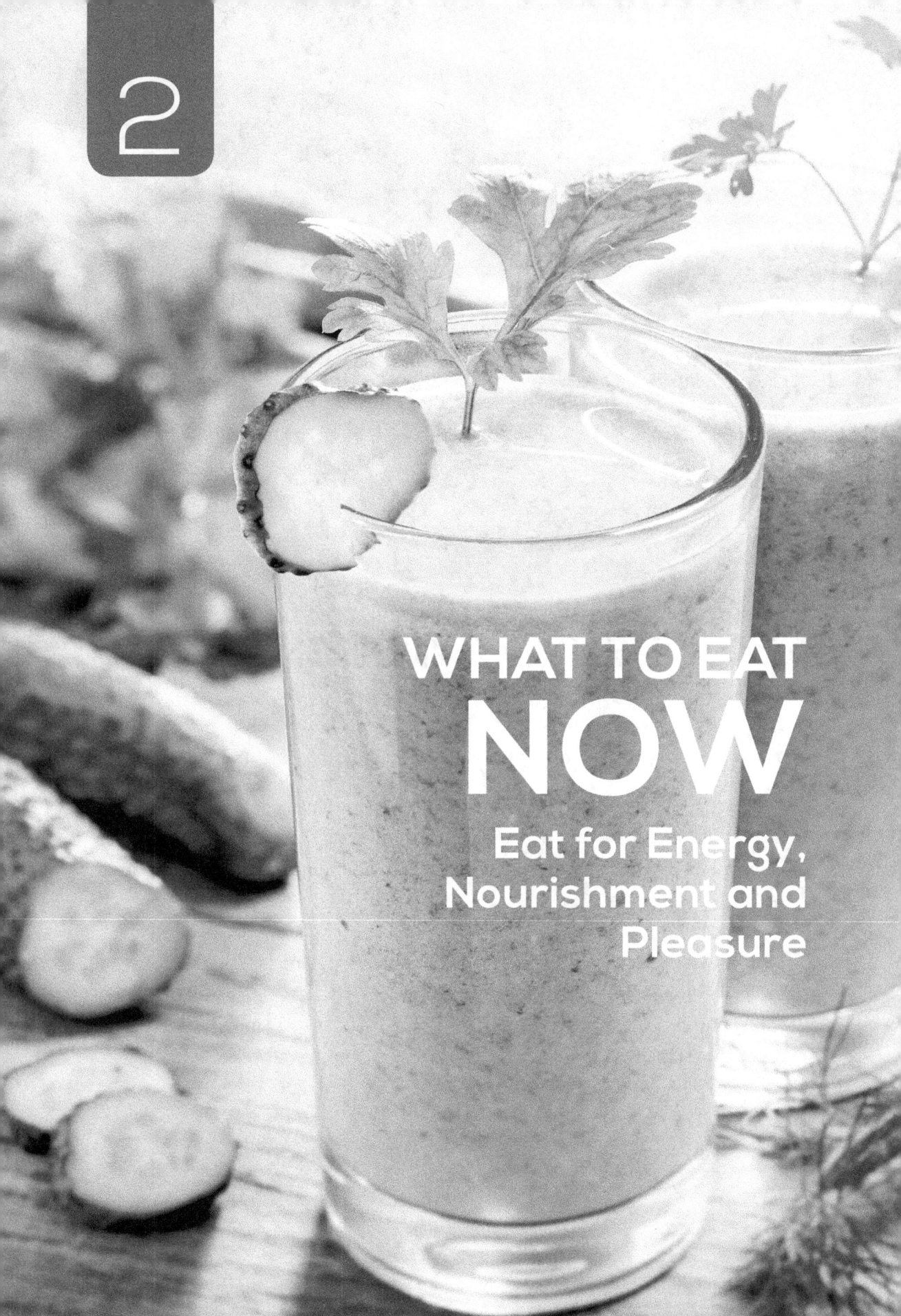

2

WHAT TO EAT NOW

Eat for Energy, Nourishment and Pleasure

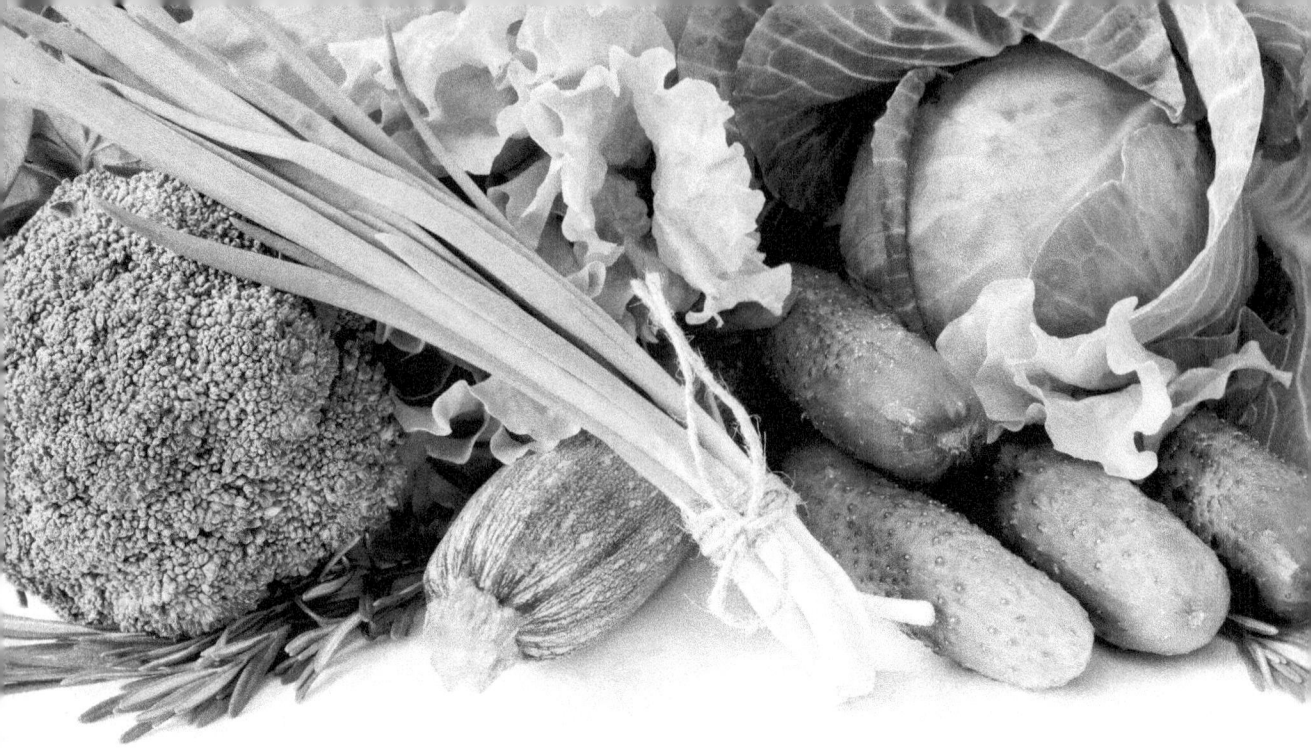

FOODS THAT WILL ENERGIZE
THE MIND AND BODY

In this chapter, you'll learn what qualifies as a nutrient dense, living food and how to incorporate more of these foods into your diet to experience more energy, and how to listen to your body and eat according to what it tells you to feel your absolute best.

So now that you know what *not* to eat, let's explore the foods that will make you feel more energetic and alive and will nourish you on all levels. I'm talking about eating nutrient dense, plant-based, living food that has been grown mindfully and responsibly.

NUTRIENT DENSE FOOD
Food to Fuel your Body and Mind

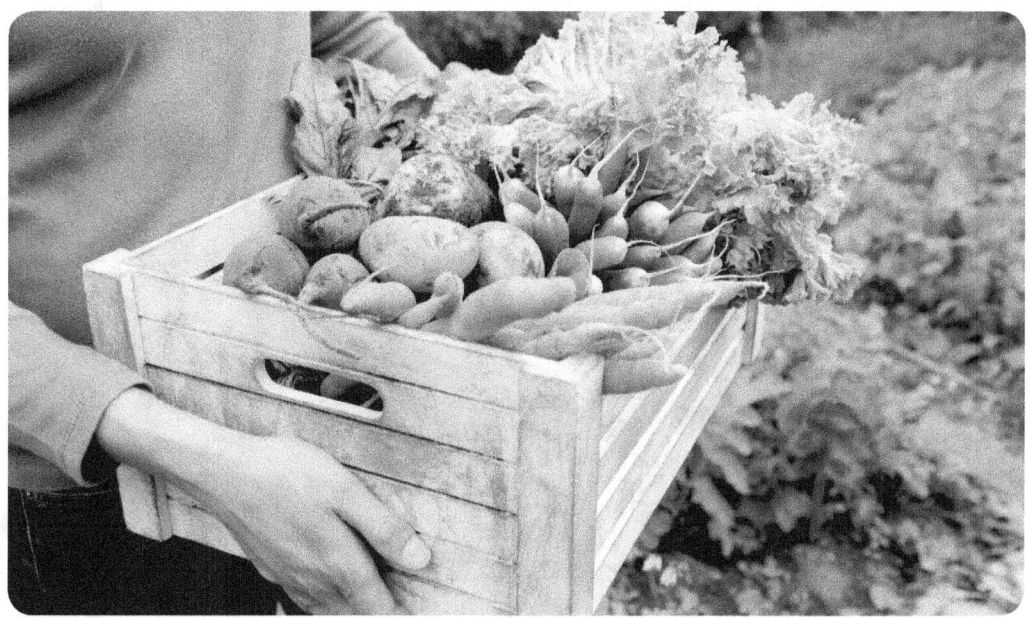

Nutrient dense living food is simply food that is high in vitamins, minerals and antioxidants. It is whole, minimally processed and **hasn't** been exposed to the dangerous farming practices you learned about in chapter 1. Nutrient dense foods will fuel your body and mind, boost your immune system and usually are much lower in calories.

Nutrient dense living foods include:
- Whole grains
- Organic fruits and vegetables
- Organic nuts, seeds and beans
- Superfoods

Nutrient Dense and Living

Living foods are foods that still contain some of the energy (life force) that once allowed them to be alive. Fruits, vegetables, and superfoods that have not been processed in any way are examples of living foods. Living food is usually not found in a can, bag, or package. The sooner you can get more living foods into your body, the better. Eating locally grown organic food is best.

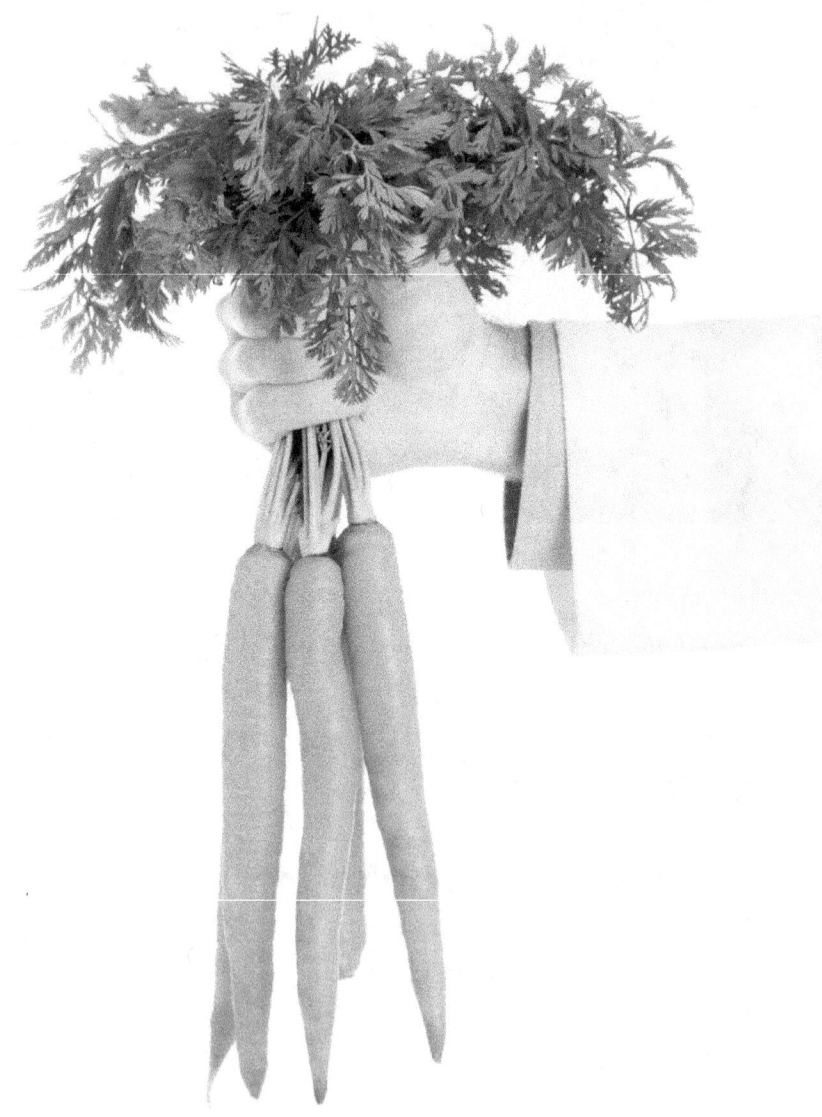

EAT PLANT-BASED

Shoot to consume as much of your food from nutrient dense plant sources as possible. This is called eating plant-based and is not only better for our planet, but also for your digestive system. Simply put, meat is hard to digest and you must expend a lot of energy to digest it. By having most of your diet come from plants, you're setting yourself up for high energy, high nutrient gain and increased body alkalinity. Body alkalinity is important to reduce inflammation in the body, which is the root of almost every chronic disease. To create an alkaline environment in your body, eat more nutrient dense, plant-based, living foods.

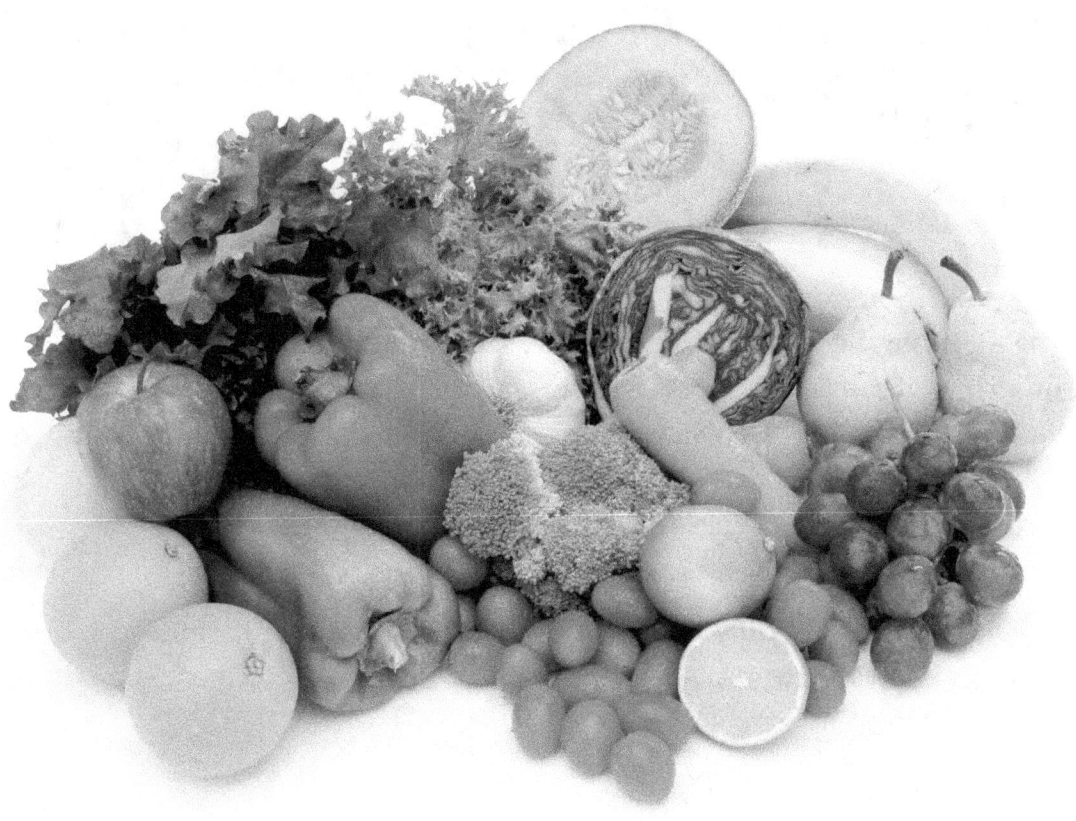

RESPONSIBLY FARMED ANIMAL PROTEIN

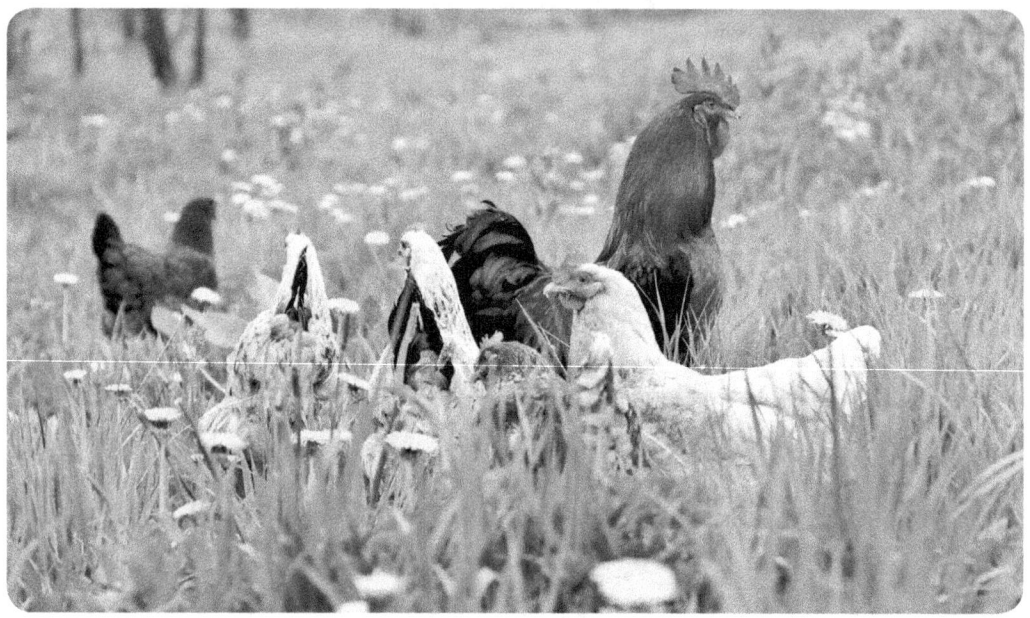

However, if you are someone who depends on animal protein, don't worry. The important thing to remember is that **it's about quality over quantity.** If eating meat works for your body, purchase the highest quality you can afford. Knowing how the animals you're eating have been raised and treated is key. Buy USDA certified organic meat products. This certification ensures the animals have been treated humanely and raised without the use of hormones and antibiotics.

Examples of responsibly farmed animal protein sources include:

- Organic grass-fed beef and bison
- Organic chicken and turkey
- Wild-caught fish

SUPERFOODS

Simply put, superfoods are the most potent nutrient rich foods on the planet. They have the ability to increase energy, detoxify the body, boost the immune system, lower inflammation and completely nourish the body at the cellular level.

The super "superfoods":
- Cacao
- Goji berries
- Spirulina
- Chlorella
- Bee pollen
- Maca
- Medicinal mushrooms (Reishi, Chaga, Cordyseps, Maitake, Shitake)
- Wheatgrass juice
- Sunflower and pea sprouts

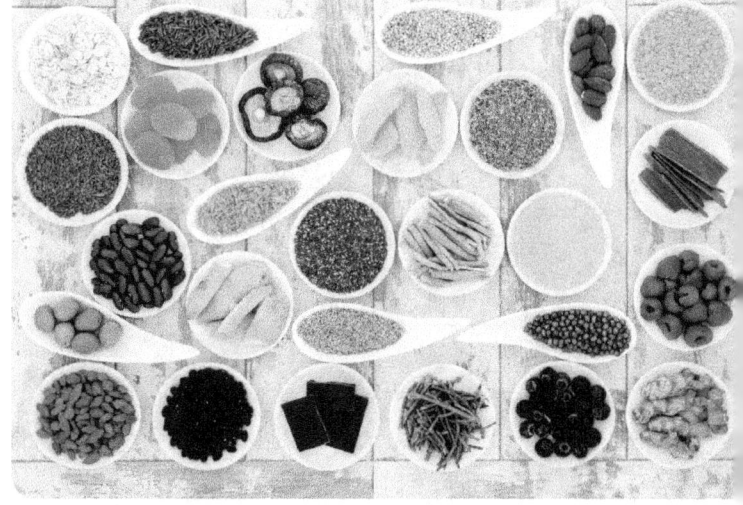

You'll find more details about each superfood listed and their amazing health properties in the supplemental materials [pgs 64-66] of this chapter. The easiest way to start incorporating superfoods into your diet is by simply preparing a superfood smoothie. Use the superfood smoothie guide [pg 67] to make easy delicious superfood combinations for nutrient packed smoothies.

ORGANIC AND LOCAL

It's so important to buy organically grown foods when and where possible. Organic foods are not processed using irradiation, not sprayed with dangerous farming chemicals, not grown in chemical fertilizers, not genetically modified, nor do they contain any chemical food additives. Purchasing organically grown food protects our water quality, saves energy, and promotes biodiversity.

Organic foods also contain more nutrients and simply taste better. But even better than buying organic food, is buying **local and organic.** The closer you eat to the place that your food was grown, the more energy and nutrients it contains.

For example: If you live in Florida and are shopping for grapefruit, which is a better choice? Purchasing an organic grapefruit grown and shipped in from New Zealand? Or buying one picked off the tree from the farm up the road? The choice is obvious, but many people overlook this crucial simple concept.

At this point, you may be wondering where you can get local and organic food. I have provided you with a natural food directory resource worksheet [pg 60] to help you find local and organic food in your area.

It's important to note that many local farmers use organic growing methods, but don't have the USDA certified organic label. Ask the farmer if they grow using organic methods when buying from local farmers markets.

BIO INDIVIDUALITY:
Listening To Your Body

We all are unique, have different body and blood types, live in different locations, have different genetics, caloric needs and lifestyles. With that being said, when it comes to eating for optimal health, **there is not a one size fits all approach to eating that works for everyone.** However, what does work for everyone is steering clear of man-made processed foods and eating more living, nutrient dense foods.

Our bodies are the most amazing machines and will send feedback signals as to what foods work best with our unique bodies, but it's up to us to "tune-in" and really listen. The healthier you become, the more sensitive you'll be to your body's wants and needs. I call this process becoming "in-tune" with the body. This doesn't happen overnight, but rather over weeks and months of eating nutrient dense living foods. Interestingly, once your "in-tune" you may find that even eating certain types of "healthy" food doesn't seem to work with your unique body. For example, you may feel tired, bloated or even anxious after eating something healthy like broccoli. Figuring out what foods really work for your body can be a very difficult process. However, the more "in-tune" and mindful you are to how you feel based on the food you eat, the easier this process becomes. By staying connected and aware of how your body is responding to the foods you're consuming (both the "healthy" and "unhealthy" foods), you'll be able to reach a higher level of energy, awareness and experience mental clarity.

The most common food sensitivities are to dairy products, gluten, soy, sugar/ artificial sweeteners, corn and peanuts. Be especially mindful of how your body responds when eating these foods...low energy level, mental fog and nasal congestion are all signs you may be sensitive to a food.

The Turning Point

The "turning point" is when your body becomes hyper-sensitive to which foods work best for your body. This usually takes place after eating clean nutrient dense living foods for several weeks and months.

Once you reach this point, it's time to use the bio-food identifier worksheet [pg 74] to really hone in on how certain types of foods (both the "good" and "not so good") effect your mood, energy level, emotions, digestion and mental clarity.

This process does take time, but is well worth the effort. Once you determine which foods truly work for your body, then you will really start to feel and experience what it's like to have optimal energy, mental clarity and extraordinary health.

*Use the bio-food identifier worksheet to determine what foods work best for your unique bio-chemistry once you reach the "turning point."

The 90/10 Rule

The 90/10 rule is a very simple, yet powerful tool that will transform your health when it's followed consistently. The rule is to get 90 percent of the food you consume from clean plant-based whole food sources and save the other 10 percent for your 'not-so-healthy' favorite foods. By following this rule, you'll be able to enjoy your favorite 'not-so-healthy foods' without feeling deprived. Again, it's all about finding your balance.

STAY HYDRATED

Staying hydrated is so important and often not emphasized enough, in my opinion. It's estimated that around three quarters of Americans experience chronic dehydration. This is bad for many reasons. Our bodies are made up of about 70% water and our muscle tissues about 80% water. Being chronically dehydrated, which occurs with as little as a **2% drop in your bodies water supply, causes low energy, lack of focus, irritability, poor digestion and an inability to regulate body temperature.**

In general, drink about half your body weight in ounces per day. If you weigh 160 lbs., that's 80 oz. or ten 8 oz. glasses of water per day. It's important to mention that the amount greatly depends on a few other factors such as your activity level, where you live, your gender and what you eat. You do absorb some water from food which attributes to your overall water intake. Fruits and vegetables contain the most water in food form. Use the color of your urine as a gauge of your hydration level. If your urine is clear and light, you're hydrated. If it's very yellow and dark, you probably need to drink more.

After you figure out how much water you should be drinking, it's important to touch on water quality. This is another often overlooked subject that is very important. Unfortunately, today **clean water is a limited resource**. Our water is loaded with chemicals such as fluoride, chlorine and many other harmful substances. Even drinking spring water out of plastic bottles isn't really optimal because plastic leaches harmful chemicals. The best way to ensure you're getting clean water is to purchase a high quality water purifying system. They range in price, but even the cheaper ones are better than using nothing at all. I also recommend buying a 16 oz. glass reusable water bottle and carrying it around with you wherever you go. Not only will this help you remember to drink, but you can be sure you're avoiding chemicals that can leach from plastics bottles and drinking from the public water fountain. That being said, it's better to stay hydrated over not drinking the most optimal clean water.

IMPORTANT NOTE: Avoid soda, fruit juice (unless freshly squeezed) and other premade sugary drinks. Sugar is corrosive to the body and leads to weight gain and diabetes. If you're used to drinking and/or addicted to these types of beverages, simply stop buying them. At first this will be challenging since sugar is an addictive substance, but if you stick with it, you'll find the craving will soon subside.

Stay optimally hydrated every day to...
- Increase energy
- Ensure optimal digestion
- Lubricate joints and muscles

*Get in the habit of drinking a glass of lemon water as soon as you wake up. Set it by your bed so you don't forget. This will not only help hydrate you, but the lemon will help balance your body's alkalinity, reducing inflammation and improving energy levels.

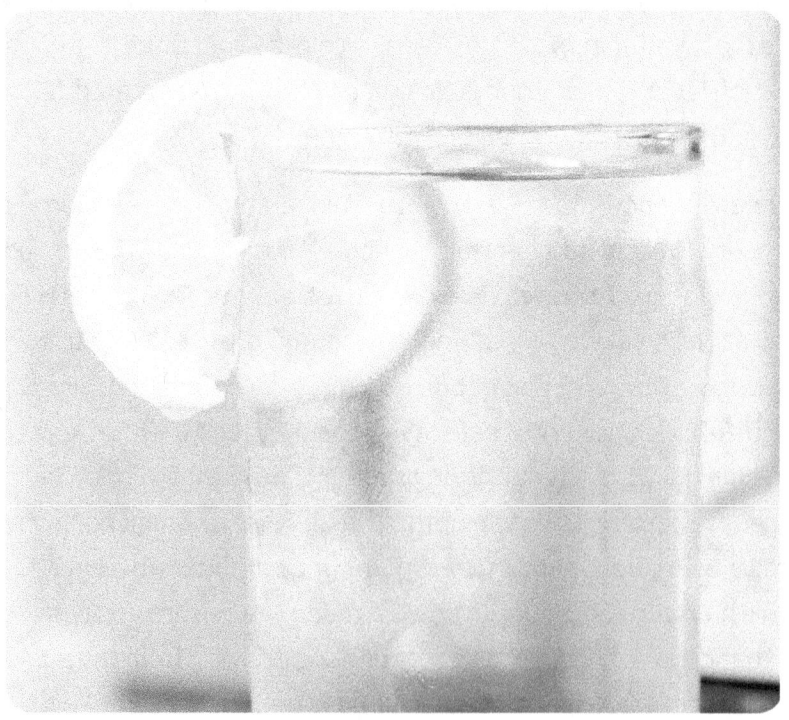

NUTRITIONAL SCIENCE 101
Macronutrients: Carbohydrates, Fats and Protein

Carbohydrates 101

Many people get confused about carbohydrates since the media and recent fad diets tell us they will make us fat. Although this can be true, it is only true if you are eating the wrong kind of carbohydrates. The anti-carb movement should really be an anti-processed carb movement. An easy way to remember a "good" carb from a "bad" is to think of them in terms of "whole verses part." Whole grains, fruits and vegetables are good carbohydrates and processed foods (refined) white pasta, white flour, white bread, candies, cookies and baked goods are bad carbs. In nutritional science, they divide carbohydrates in two categories, complex (think whole, good) and simple (processed, bad with the exception of fruit).

What is a whole grain? A whole grain is the entire grain, which includes the bran, germ and endosperm. Whole grains have been a central element of the human diet since early civilization. Once harvested, these grains have a very long shelf-life, providing energy during harsh seasons when fresh fruits and vegetables were scarce. Whole grains are an excellent source of nutrition, as they contain essential enzymes, iron, dietary fiber, vitamin E and B-complex vitamins. Because the body absorbs grains slowly, they provide sustained and high-quality energy.

So, how many good carbs should you be eating a day? This depends on your lifestyle, age, gender, weight and health goals. My simple strategy is eat as much vegetables as you'd like and include whole grains in your daily diet. Avoid simple processed carbs.

Examples of Good Carbohydrates:

Whole Grains: brown rice, buckwheat (aka kasha), oats (whole groats), oatmeal (rolled oats), amaranth, barley, bulgur (cracked wheat), cornmeal (aka polenta), couscous, kamut, millet, quinoa, rye berries, spelt, wheat berries, wild rice.

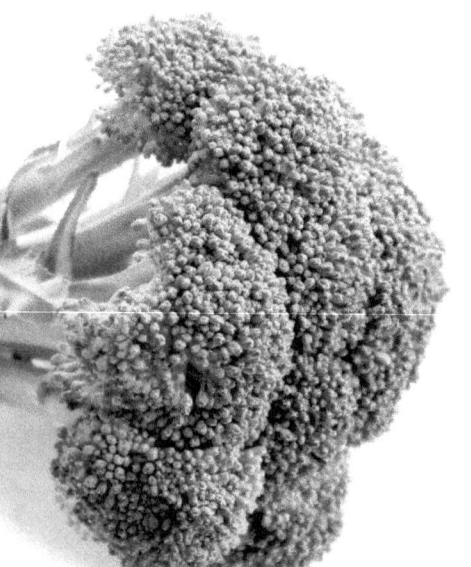

Vegetables: spinach, zucchini, asparagus, okra, celery, cucumbers, broccoli, brussels sprouts, eggplant, sweet potatoes, onions.

Fruit: Grapefruit, apples, oranges, pears, plums, carrots, strawberries, blueberries.

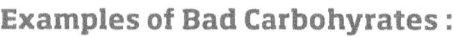

Examples of Bad Carbohyrates :

Table sugar, corn syrup, fruit juice (unless freshly squeezed), candy, cake, white bread, white pasta, soda, baked goods made with white flour, most packaged cereals, processed foods.

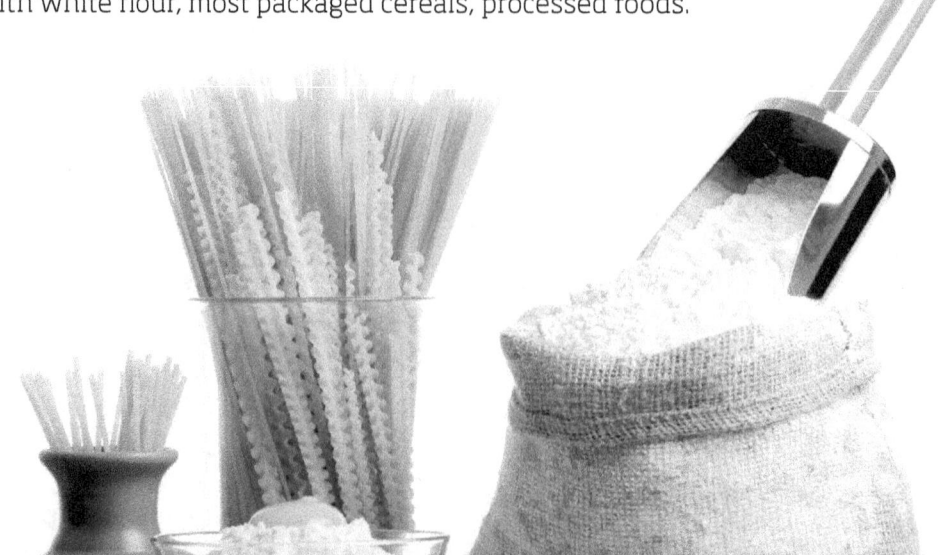

Carbohydrates and the Glycemic Index Simplified

Simply put, the Glycemic Index (GI) is a system that ranks carbohydrate-containing foods on a scale from 1 to 100 based on their effect on blood-sugar levels. A lower number (lower GI) means a lower impact on your blood sugar levels, which is a good thing. Fat and fiber also lower the GI of a food. Generally, the more processed a food is, the higher the GI.

- Low GI foods (55 or less)
- Medium GI (55-69)
- High GI (70 or more)

Why Glycemic Index is important.
Low GI diets have been associated with **decreased risk** of cardiovascular disease, type 2 diabetes, metabolic syndrome, stroke, depression, chronic kidney disease, formation of gall stones, neural tube defects, formation of uterine fibroids, and cancers of the breast, colon, prostate and pancreas. [1]

Glycemic Index & vegetables (complex carbohydrates)
Low GI
Carrots, eggplant, garlic, green peas, onions, winter squash, avocados, bell papers, cucumbers, kale, mushrooms, tomatoes, celery
Moderate GI
Beets, corn, leeks, sweet potatoes
High GI
Potatoes

Glycemic Index & fruits (healthy simple carbohydrates)

Low GI

All berries (raspberries, blueberries, strawberries)

Moderate GI

Melons, grapefruit, pear, orange, lemons, peaches, apples, limes, avocados, plums

High GI

Banana, mango, pineapple, grapes, watermelon, papaya

Glycemic Index & whole grains (complex carbohyrates)

Low GI

Barley, brown rice, buckwheat, oats, quinoa, rye, whole wheat

Moderate GI

Millet

High GI

N/A

Glycemic Index & legumes aka beans (complex carbohyrates)

Low GI

Soybeans, tofu, tempeh, black beans, garbanzo beans, kidney beans, lentil, lima bean, navy, beans, pinto beans

Moderate GI

N/A

High GI

N/A

---

[1] The world's healthiest foods. "What is the Glycemic Index?" Discussion.
www.whfoods.com , N.P., 2014 Web.

Protein is the basic building block for the human structure. It makes up our muscles, tissues, skin and hair. Protein is essential to a healthy diet and life.

There are many factors that determine what the right amount of protein is best for our individual bodies. However, age, gender and activity level are a good place to start. For example, young active males need more protein than middle aged women who are moderately active. The best way to determine how much protein is right for you is to experiment with different amounts and sources and see how your body responds. The amount could be more or less depnding on your lifestyle and goals. Most Americans eat way too much protein. Figuring out the right amount of protein for your body takes some trial and error but it's worth the trouble. Try both plant and animal protein sources of the **highest quality**. Start with keeping protein portions to the size of your palm or smaller and go from there.

History and Challenges of Animal Protein Consumption:

For centuries, many cultures have been eating animal protein: Eskimos, Native Americans, Africans, Europeans, Chinese, and even the Tibetans. However, there are many issues associated with the production and consumption of animal protein. Unfortunately, most of our meat comes from factory farming. Factory farmed animals are treated with great cruelty. They are injected with growth hormones and antibiotics and fed unnaturally to be massed produced for maximum profits. It's important to eat high-quality, organic, free-range, grass fed forms of animal protein whenever possible. Remember if the animal is healthy, you will in turn be healthy.

*To make animal protein easier to digest, eat plenty of vegetables with your meal. The enzymes released from the plants will help break down the protein.

Nourishing Animal Protein Sources

Chicken, turkey, buffalo, grass fed beef, eggs and wild caught fish .

Fishy Fish: Fish farming is now a huge business. Farmed fish are generally fed unnatural feed to increase their size, injected with coloring for consumer buying appeal, and given antibiotics to prevent disease due to overcrowding. Often they also contain high levels of mercury, which is toxic to humans. If you choose to eat fish, eat wild-caught fish when possible.

Nourishing Plant Sources of Protein

Whole grains: Brown rice, buckwheat (aka kasha), oats (whole groats), amaranth, barley, bulgur (cracked wheat), and quinoa.

Beans: Lentils, black beans, chickpeas, kidney beans, mung beans, adzuki beans. Beans contain a more complete set of amino acids than other plant foods. If you're not used to eating beans, eat fresh smaller beans such as split peas, mung or adzuki beans for they are easier to digest. Also, soaking them overnight, adding spices or vinegar, skimming off the cooking foam, pressure cooking and puréeing them will help with digestion of beans.

Nuts: Peanuts, almonds, walnuts, cashews.
Generally considered a fat, not a protein. Nuts are great for people who want to gain weight. Peanuts, which are actually legumes (beans), are far higher in protein than any "nuts". Go organic when buying peanut products to avoid GMO peanuts and trans-fats.

Seeds: Savi seeds, hemp seeds, pumpkin seeds.

Fat 101

There is a considerable amount of conflicting stories in the media about fat. It's no wonder people are confused about which fats are healthy and which are not. I'm going to keep it very simple. There are four main types of fats. Saturated, monounsaturated, polyunsaturated, and trans-fatty acids. Let's break them down.

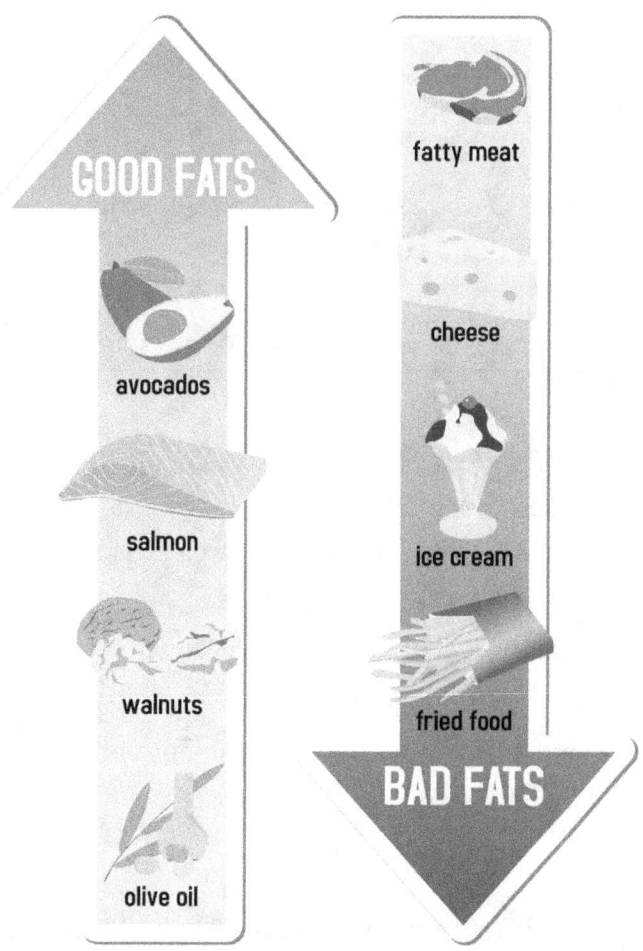

GOOD FATS
- avocados
- salmon
- walnuts
- olive oil

BAD FATS
- fatty meat
- cheese
- ice cream
- fried food

GOOD FATS vs. BAD FATS

Bad Fats:

1. **Saturated**: Consumption of long chain fatty acids (LCFAs) can increase risk of heart disease. **Eat in moderation**.
   Found in beef, chicken, turkey, pork, cow's milk, palm oil, and full fat dairy products; e.g., yogurt.
2. **Trans-fat**: Raises bad cholesterol (LDL), lowers good (HDL). Increases risk of chronic diseases. **Avoid entirely**!
   Found in margarine, processed foods, candy, chips, soda, processed baked goods and some peanut butters.

Good Fats:

1. **Monounsaturated**: Raises good cholesterol (HDL) and lowers bad cholesterol (LDL). **Eat often**.
   Found in avocados, olives, olive oil, nuts, seeds, fish, and some vegetables.
2. **Polyunsaturated**: Raises good cholesterol (HDL), lowers bad cholesterol (LDL), anti-inflammatory. **Eat often**.
   Found in fish, flax seeds, and walnuts.
3. **Saturated**: Medium chain triglycerides (MCTs) are sent directly to your liver, where they are converted into energy rather than stored as fat. **Eat often**.
   Found in coconut.

Polyunsaturated fats contain Omega 3, 6, 9 fatty acids. Omega 3, 6, 9 fatty acids are different types of polyunsaturated fats, which have different affects on the body. Here is a simple break down and where they can be found.

Omega-3:
Essential fatty acid, which means our bodies don't make them. Includes beneficial fatty acids EPA, DHA and linoleic acid.
Found in herring, sardines, mackerel, salmon, chia seeds, and micro-algae (spirulina, chlorella).

Omega-6:
Essential fatty acid, which means our bodies don't make them. Includes beneficial fatty acids, linoleic fatty acid and arachidonic acid.
Found in avocado, durum wheat, flaxseed oil, hemp oil, soybean oil, acai berry, and cashews.

Omega-9:

Not essential because our bodies make this type. Includes oleic acid, erucic acid, elaidic acid, eicosenoic acid, mead acid, and nervonic acid.

Found in olive oil, rapeseed oil, and mustard seed.

Best oils for cooking:

* Smoke point = the temperature oil can be heated before it starts decomposing. Use oils with a smoke point at or above 400 degree F when cooking at high temperatures.

- Pure olive oil (not extra virgin) smoke point 438 degree F
- Grapeseed oil smoke point 420 degree F
- Virgin (unrefined) coconut oil smoke point 350 degree F
- Expeller-pressed canola oil smoke point 400 degree F
- Avocado oil smoke point 520 degree F

Refined vs unrefined oil:

- Refined oils are extracted using heat and a solvent, then are bleached and deodorized. These oils are best used for high tempature cooking because of their high smoke point. However they don't contain as many health benefits due to the processing method.

- Unrefined oils are cold-pressed by a machine which applies pressure rather than heat. This processing method leaves in tact the health promoting antioxidants and phytochemicals. Unrefined oils are best used during low/medium tempature cooking methods such as sauteing and used raw.

Fat is essential to a healthy diet and life. Include mono and poly unsaturated fat rich foods into your diet. Fat provides energy and enables the transport and storage of fat soluble vitamin K, A, D, and E. Fat provides insulation and a protective cover to vital organs, it is good for our hair, skin and cognitive function.

It's important to know a little bit about calories, what they are, where they come from and how they affect your body. A calorie is simply a unit of energy. Protein, carbohydrates and fats all contain calories but in different amounts per gram. Protein and carbohydrates contain 4 calories per gram and fat contains 9 calories per gram. Notice how fat has more than double the amount of calories per gram than protein and carbohydrates. This is why eating a diet consisting of a lot of fat can lead to quick weight gain. Simply put, when you eat more calories than you burn off, you gain weight usually in the form of fat. For this reason, **it's essential to know how many calories you're consuming a day and how to properly manage the amounts of calories going in and calories going out.**

The Cause	The Result	What Happens
More calories in than out	Caloric abundance	Gain fat, muscle or both
Calories in = calories out	Maintenance	Weight stays the same
Less calories in than out	Caloric deficit	Lose muscle, fat or both

After tracking the amount of calories most people consume in a day, they are usually greatly surprised at the total daily amount. This is because calories add up very fast and can be hidden in many foods. But **what's even more surprising to people is when they realize how much energy it actually takes to burn these calories off.** For example, let's say you weigh 155 pounds. You'd need to run for about 26 minutes to burn off the calories you consumed from eating a Snickers bar according to a Harvard Medical School study.

For optimal health, you'll want to stay within your daily calorie range to maintain a healthy weight. I am not a huge fan of counting calories. However, if you're overweight, to get an idea of how many calories you're consuming, you'll need to track you're daily caloric intake for at least a week. Use the calorie tracker worksheet and formula [pg 76-78] to determine about how many calories you should be consuming to reach your ideal weight and health goals.

Note: Most processed foods are loaded with calories. By simply cooking and eating real food, you'll be consuming fewer calories, especially if your diet consists of plant-based foods which generally are much less calorically dense.

An easy-to-follow rule of thumb: About one-fourth of a medium-sized plate should be devoted to a starch (complex carbohydrate), another one-fourth of the plate to a lean protein (wild fish, organic poultry, beans) and the remaining half to fruits and vegetables. However, fruit is best eaten in between meals for optimal digestablity.

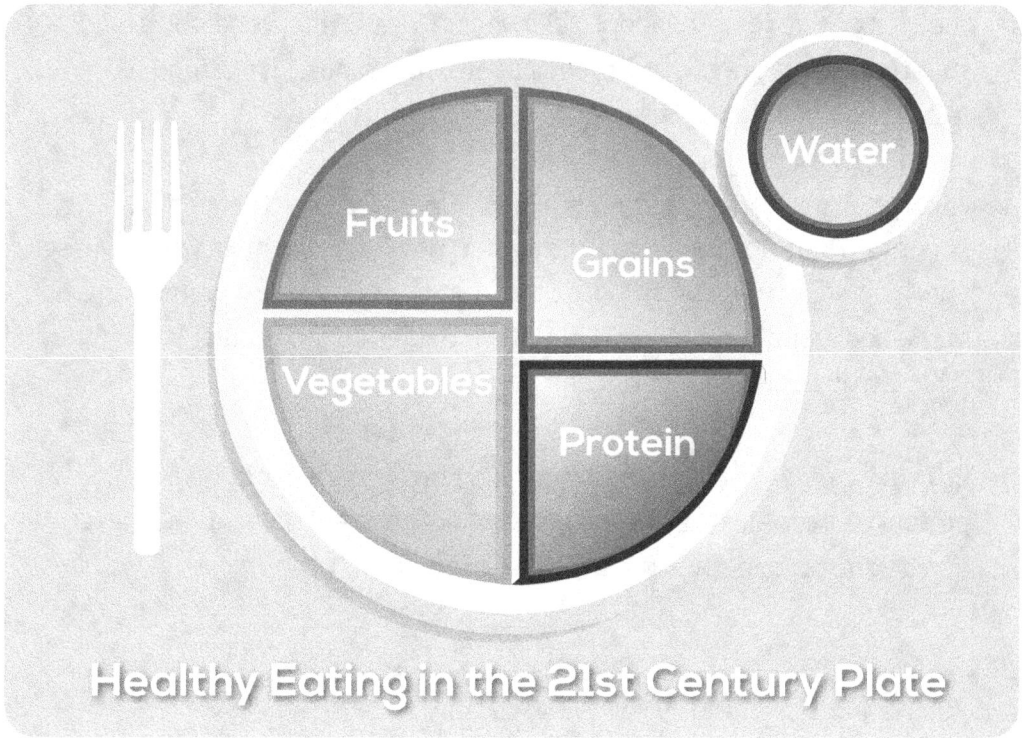

Healthy Eating in the 21st Century Plate

Key Concepts

---

1. Eat nutrient dense, plant-based, living food that has been grown mindfully and responsibly. Buying organic food when and where possible eliminates the risks of the current dangers of our modern food production methods.

2. Go plant-based. Going plant-based simply means that your diet consist of mostly food from nutrient dense plant sources. It's better for the environment and for you.

3. Living foods are those that were once alive and still contain some of the energy (life force) that once allowed it to be. Fruits, vegetables, and superfoods that are not processed are all living foods. Living food is not found in a can, bag, or package.

4. Incorporate superfoods into your diet. Superfoods are the most potent super nutrient rich foods on the planet. They have the ability to increase energy, detoxify the body, boost the immune system, lower inflammation in the body, and completely nourish our bodies at the cellular level, which is where true health is experienced.

5. Eat wild-caught fish, and antibiotic and hormone free (organic) animal protein sources. The better the quality of life the animal had, the better the quality the protein, thus the healthier for you.

6. Listen to your body and eat according to what it tells you. There is no one size fits all diet. Choose living, nutrient dense foods that work for you.

7. Good carbohydrates, fats and the right amount of protein are essential to looking and feeling your absolute best. The right ratio of macro nutrients depends on your lifestyle, age, gender, height and activity level.

8. Calories are a measurement of energy. They are found in proteins, carbohydrates and fats. It's important to know your daily caloric needs to maintain an optimal weight.

9. An easy-to-follow rule of thumb: One-fourth of a medium-sized plate should be devoted to a starch (complex carb), another one-fourth of the plate to a lean protein (wild fish, organic poultry, beans) and the remaining half to fruits and vegetables. However, fruit is best eaten in between meals for optimal digestablity.

10. Carbohydrates are the body's main source of energy. They are mainly found in starchy foods like grains, vegetables, and fruits but also can be found in dairy products, beans, nuts and seeds. Protein is the building blocks of cells, tissues, hormones. It is essential for growth and is found in meats, fish, dairy products, nuts, beans, whole grains and vegetables. Fat is needed for normal growth and development, absorbing certain vitamins (K, A, D, E) and also provides energy. Fat is found in meat, poultry, nuts, dairy products, butters and oils.

Action Items

✔ Use the health food directory worksheet [pg 60] to research in your area where to buy locally grown, organic food. Support local farmers where and when possible. Buy "Certified Organic" - it's worth it! If you don't have access or can't afford it, at the very least, try to buy the most contaminated produce items [pg 31] organic.

✔ Start incorporating more nutrient dense living foods into your diet. Real food is nutrient dense, plant-based and living. Use the essential food list [pg 113] as a shopping guide. Be an informed shopper by knowing how it was grown or treated by reading labels.

✔ Choose a few superfoods to start incorporating into your diet right away. Reference the superfood list [pg 64] for a list of the most powerful superfoods. Try making a superfood smoothie. Use the guide to superfood smoothie's worksheet [pg 67] to help you get started.

✔ Use the bio-food identifier worksheet [pgs 74-75] to determine what foods work best with your unique bio-chemistry.

✔ Calculate your water intake by dividing body weight by two. This is the about the amount you should be drinking. For example: 160 lbs. divided by 2 is 80 oz. of water per day or ten 8 oz. glasses. Purchase and use a quality water filter and a reusable glass or aluminum water bottle.

✔ Review the nutrition 101 carbs, protein and fat information [pg45-53] to fully grasp this valuable information and to understand the basic science behind the food we eat.

✔ Calculate your daily caloric needs using the "Determine How Many Calories to Consume" worksheet [pg 76]. Then track your caloric intake for 1 week using the "Calorie Tracker" worksheet [pg 78].

CHAPTER 2:
SUPPLEMENTAL MATERIALS

Natural Food Website Directory

Listing of small, individually owned health food stores:
www.greenpeople.org/healthfood.htm

Listing of natural food stores and restaurants nationally and globally:
www.happycow.net

Find a natural foods co-op near you:
www.coopdirectory.org

Find a health food store in your area:
www.vegetarianusa.com/downloadcity.html

Find organic and natural food stores:
www.organicstorelocator.com

Find food co-ops and health food stores:
www.organicconsumers.org/purelink.html

Find a Whole Foods Market in your area:
www.wholefoodsmarket.com

1. **Keep chemicals off your plate**. Pesticides are poisons designed to kill living organisms and thus are harmful to humans. Many approved pesticides were registered long before extensive research linked these chemicals to cancer and other diseases. Organic agriculture is a way to prevent any more of these chemicals from getting into the air, water and food supply.

2. **Protect future generations**. Children are four times more sensitive to exposure to cancer-causing pesticides in foods than adults. Cancer rates are going through the roof. Do you know someone or have you been personally affected by cancer? If you answered 'yes,' you're not alone. Today 1 out of every 3 people will be diagnosed with some kind of cancer.

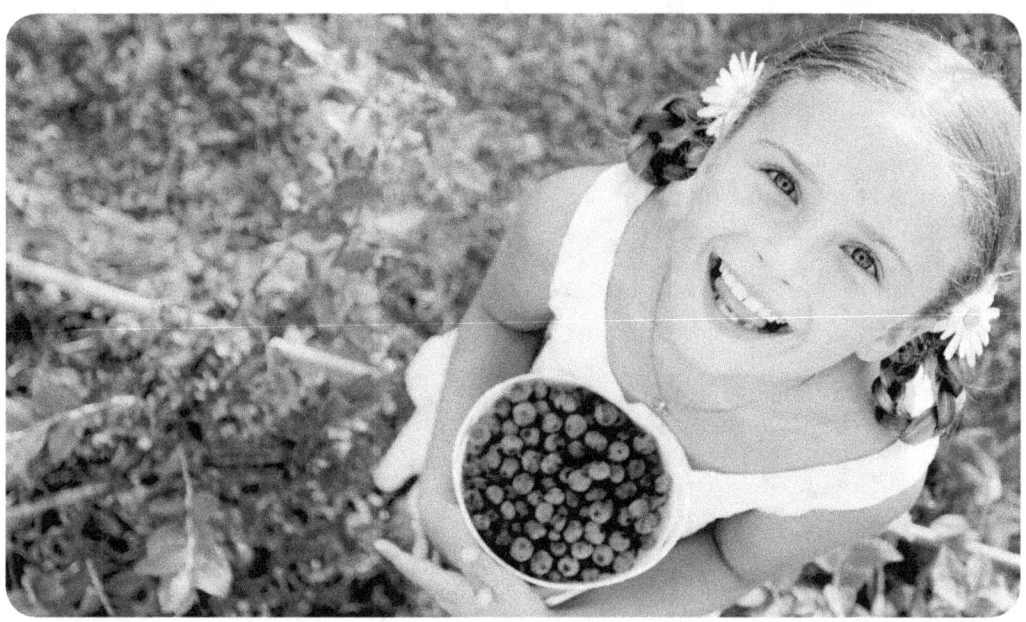

3. **Protect water quality**. Pesticides pollute the public's primary source of drinking water for more than half the country's population. Unfortunately, fresh clean water is now a limited resource.

4. **Organic farmers work in harmony with nature**. Three billion tons of topsoil erodes from crop lands in the U.S. each year, and much of it is due to conventional farming practices, which often ignore the health of the soil, which is where all the nutrients in our food are produced. Organic agriculture respects the balance necessary for a healthy ecosystem.

5. **Save energy**. More energy is now used to produce synthetic fertilizers than to till, cultivate and harvest all the crops in the U.S. The industrial mono crop farming practices in the U.S. are not sustainable.

6. **Help small farmers**. Although more and more large-scale farms are making the conversion to organic practices, most organic farms are small, independently owned and operated family businesses. The USDA reported that in 1997, half of U.S. farm production came from only 2% of farms. Organic agriculture can be a lifeline for small farms because it offers an alternative market where sellers can demand fair prices for crops.

7. **Support a true economy**. Organic foods might seem expensive at first. However, your tax dollars pay for hazardous waste clean-up and environmental damage caused by conventional farming, so in reality we would be saving money if we made a shift back to organic farming practices, not to mention you'd personally be saving money in the long run by avoiding paying expensive medical bills from getting sick. There was a study done that showed for every dollar you spend on your health now you save three dollars later.

8. **Promote biodiversity**. Planting large plots of land with the same crop (also known as mono crop farming) year after year tripled farm production between 1950 and 1970, but the lack of natural diversity of plant life has negatively affected soil quality.

9. **Nourishment and nutrients**. Organic farming starts with the nourishment of the soil, and in turn, produces nourishing plants with more nutrients than conventionally grown produce.

10. **Flavor**. Many people find that organic produce simply tastes better. Try it and see for yourself.

Superfoods are the most potent super nutrient rich foods on the planet. They have the ability to increase energy, detoxify the body, boost the immune system, lower inflammation in the body and completely nourish our bodies at the cellular level, which is where true healing takes place. Below are the superstars of the superfoods. Start to incorporate some of these foods into your daily dietary lifestyle. An easy way to do this is by supplementing your diet with plant-based smoothies with a few of these added in. Today you can find these amazing superfoods online or at almost any natural health food store.

1. **Cacao (raw chocolate)** contains the world's highest concentration of antioxidants in the world and is the #1 source of magnesium, iron, manganese and chromium. It improves cardiovascular health, builds strong bones and is a natural mood elevator. In many cultures, cacao is considered a sacred food.

2. **Goji berries** are the most nutritionally rich berry on the planet, 4 times more potent than blueberries. This berry is not only full of vitamins and trace minerals, but it is a complete protein source containing all 9 essential amino acids. This is why it has been used in traditional Chinese medicine for over 5,000 years. Goji berries contain zinc, iron, copper, calcium, germanium, selenium, phosphorus and vitamins B1, B2, B6 and E.

3. **Camu camu berries** contain the highest vitamin C source on the planet: 60 times more per serving than an orange. This berry is great for enhancing energy and the immune system. It contains an array of antioxidants and has been known to support cognitive function.

4. **Spirulina** is fresh water, single celled, spiral shaped, blue-green algae. It has the highest concentration of complete bioavailable protein (by weight) of any known food (65%). It provides a vast array of minerals, trace elements, phytonutrients and enzymes to support optimal health. It is a rich source of vitamin A, B1, B2, B6, E and K. It contains gamma-linoleic acid (GLA), which is an anti-inflammatory and nervous system essential.

5. **Chlorella** is a fresh water, single-celled, circle-shaped, green algae. It boosts the highest source of chlorophyll per gram than any other plant. It also is a complete protein (60%) by weight. It is also full of immune system and energy-boosting vitamins and minerals. It contains chlorella growth factor (CGF) which increases tissue repair, supports probiotic growth and fights free-radicals (cancer causing cells). It is a rich source of vitamin A, B1, B2, B6, E and K.

6. **Bee products**: Bee pollen is one of the most complete foods found in nature. It contains nearly all the B vitamins and 21 essential amino acids, making it a complete protein. Honey in its raw state is a rich source of minerals, antioxidants, probiotics and enzymes.

7. **Maca:** This sacred root has been cultivated in the high Peruvian Andes for thousands of years. It's known for its adaptogenic effects of increasing energy, libido, strength and endurance. Look for maca that has been gelatinized. This process makes it more concentrated and easier to digest and absorb than raw maca powder.

8. **Medicinal mushrooms (Reishi, Chaga, Cordyseps, Maitake, Shitake)** have been proven to help heal cancer and a variety of other diseases. They have super immune enhancing components.

9. **Wheatgrass juice** has the nutritional value of 2 ½ lbs of leafy green vegetables per oz. Freshly juiced wheat grass is 70% chlorophyll, which is an amazing blood detoxifier/cleanser. It is so nutrient dense (full of bioavailable vitamins, minerals, antioxidants and amino acids), that you could survive on wheat grass alone for quite some time. In fact, it is so powerful it's used in some alternative cancer therapies.

10. **Sunflower and pea sprouts** sprouts contain 10-30 times the nutrient concentration of adult size vegetables. This is because when a seed is germinated, it releases essential enzymes, vitamins, minerals and amino acids until it can draw these life giving components from the soil to grow. Sunflower and pea sprouts are also complete protein sources containing all 9 essential amino acids.

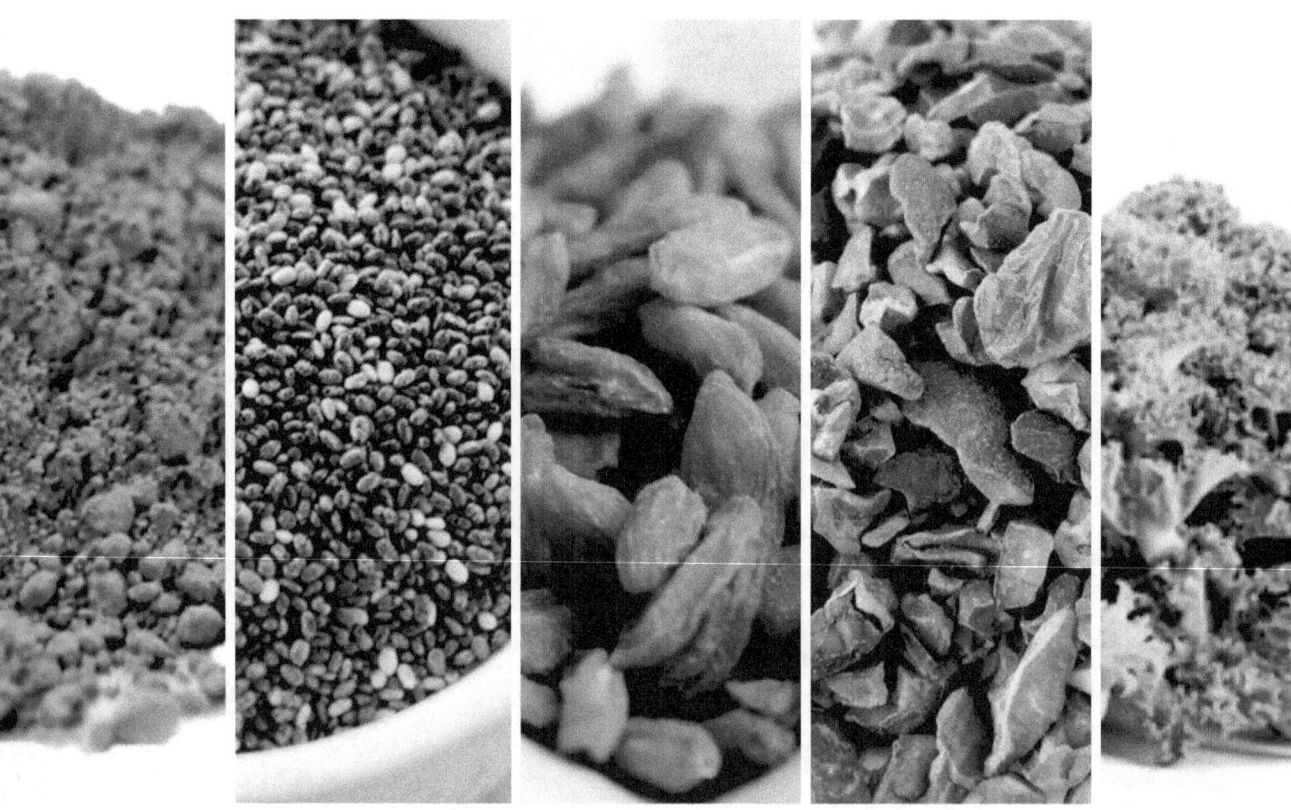

There's more than one way to make a delicious and nutrient packed superfood smoothie. The combinations are seemingly endless. Try simply choosing at least one ingredient from each column on page 68, blend and enjoy.

Tips:

- Ripe, frozen bananas make a great smoothie base (be sure to peel them before you put them in the freezer. They add a sweet flavor and creamy texture. Try using one banana and half a cup of other fruit.
- If you're not accustomed to eating many greens, try starting with 1 cup instead of 2, but be sure to use a whole cup of liquid.
- If you don't have a high-powered blender (like a Vitamix or Blendtec), try blending the liquid and greens together before adding the frozen fruit. This will ensure a smooth consistency and make the mixture easier to blend.
- Use as many superfood add-ins as you like.
- This chart is not meant to be an exhaustive list of all possible smoothie ingredients. Once you've mastered a few basic smoothies, don't be afraid to experiment.

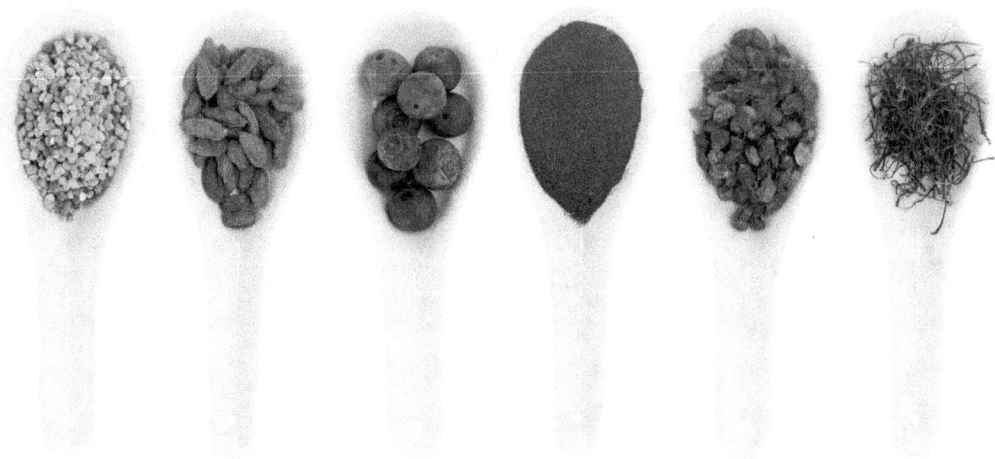

1 cup liquid	1-2 cups greens	1 cup fresh or frozen fruit	Add-ins
Flax milk	Spinach	Banana	Nut butters (almond, cashew, peanut, sunflower)
Almond milk	Kale	Cherries (pitted)	Cacao or carob powder
Coconut milk	Swiss chard	Blueberries	Vanilla bean
Coconut water	Romaine, leaf lettuce	Strawberries, raspberries, blackberries	Plant based protein powder (hemp, pea, brown rice)
100% Pressed apple juice	Turnip, beet, collard, dandelion greens	Mango, pineapple, papaya	Gelatinized maca powder, chia seeds, goji berries, acai berries, bee-pollen, raw or manduka honey
Hemp milk	Parsley	Peach, plum, pear	Cinnamon, flax seeds, chia seeds, kelp, spirulina, chlorella, green tea, aloe

Superfood smoothie recipes to get you started...

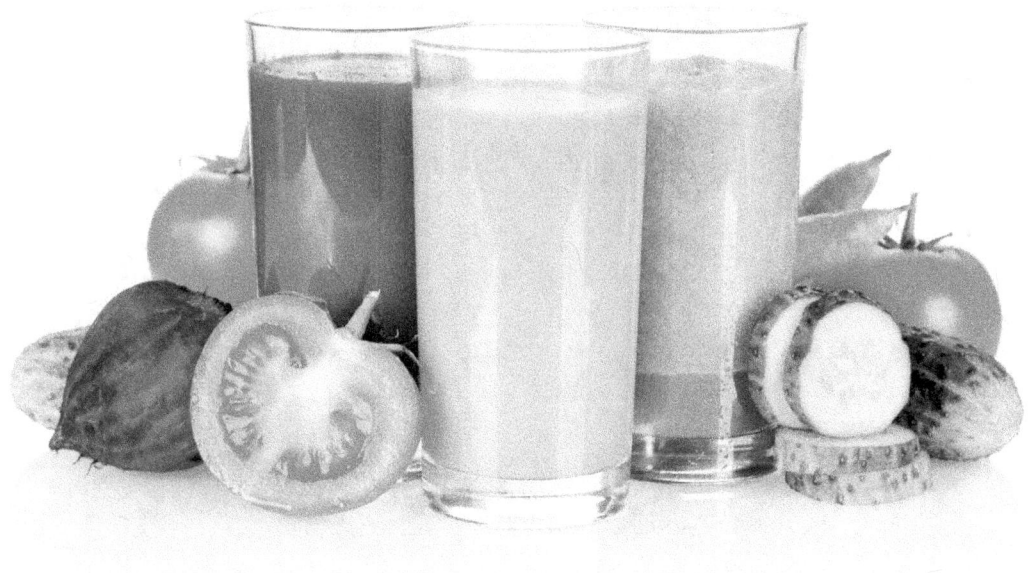

The Superfood Sensation Smoothie:

1 cup unsweetened plain or vanilla almond milk or flax milk

2 cups organic baby spinach, 1 tsp spirulina, 1 tsp chlorella

1 whole frozen banana (peel before freezing)

¼ cup frozen organic wild blueberries

¼ cup frozen organic raspberries

1 scoop plant based protein powder (hemp, pea, brown rice)

The G Bomb Energy Smoothie:

1 cup water
8 oz yerba mate
¼ cup organic frozen strawberries
¼ cup frozen organic wild blueberries
1 tsp chia seeds
½ frozen banana (peel before freezing)
1 scoop plant based protein powder (hemp, pea, brown rice)
2 cups organic baby spinach
1 tsp manduka 16+ honey

Pina-Chlorella Smoothie:

1 cup coconut water
1/2 cup fresh or frozen pineapple chunks
1/3 small avocado
1 tsp chlorella
1 tsp chia seeds or chia seed gel
1 tsp maca
1 tsp bee pollen
Squeeze of lemon juice, about 1 tsp
Optional: dash of Himalayan pink salt , a little raw honey

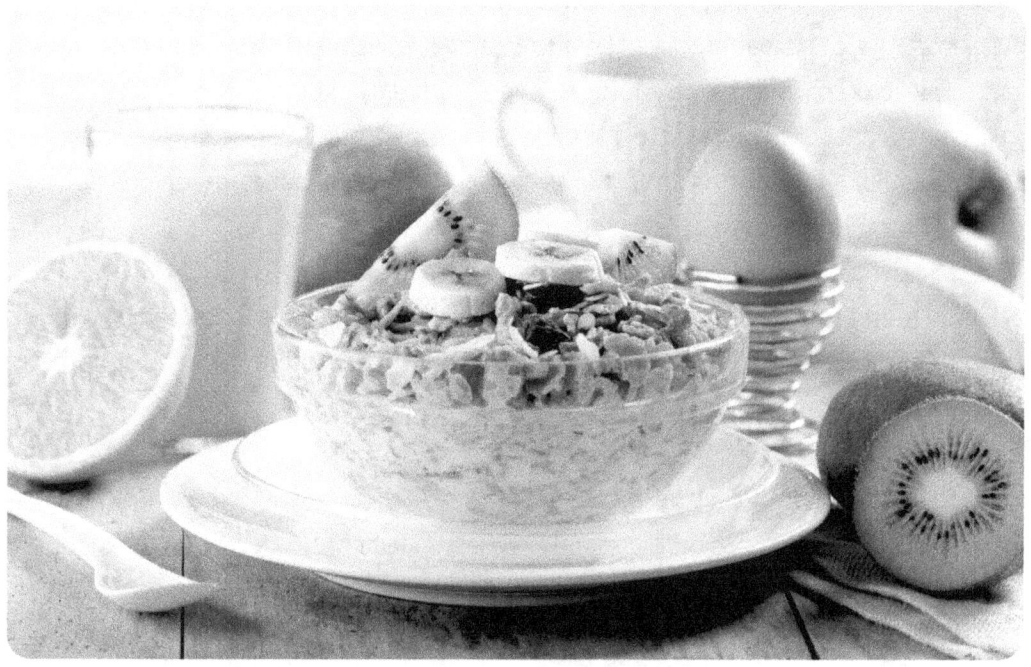

Good Sources of Protein (lean muscle building):

Organic chicken (without skin), organic turkey (without skin), lean cuts of grass fed beef, lean cuts of lamb, organic eggs, wild-caught fish (tuna, salmon, flounder, snapper, trout), unsweetened almond milk, unsweetened flax milk, black beans, garbanzo beans (aka chick peas), kidney beans, lentils, white beans, pinto beans, miso, non GMO soybeans, peanuts, almonds, cashews, hazelnuts, pecans, pistachio nuts, quinoa, natural peanut butter, almond butter, sunflower seed butter, pumpkin seeds, sunflower seeds, plant-based protein powder.

Good Sources of Carbohydrates (energy foods):

Quinoa, brown rice, 100% whole-grain bread, 100% whole grain pita bread, whole wheat/whole grain pasta, bean pasta, sweet potatoes, yams, oatmeal (steal cut), buckwheat, bulgur, bran based cereals, garbanzo beans (aka chick peas), kidney beans, black beans, lentils, navy beans, pinto beans, couscous, farro.

Fruits and Vegetables (the greener the vegetable the better):

Apple, orange, plum, banana, grapes, strawberries, peaches, pears, cantaloupe, pineapple, broccoli, brussels sprouts, cabbage, asparagus, spinach, spring lettuce, kale, swiss chard, rainbow chard, romaine lettuce, avocado, cucumber, eggplant, tomato, cauliflower, celery, turnip, bok choy, mushrooms, peppers, green peas.

Good Sources of Fat (good for the heart and brain):

Salmon, mackerel, herring, halibut, organic peanuts, almonds, cashews, almond butter, sunflower seed butter, olive oil (extra-virgin), flax seeds, flax seed oil, pumpkin seeds, chia seeds, chia oil, sunflower seeds, coconut oil.

Superfoods (make you superhuman):

Cacao (raw chocolate), goji berries, camu berries, spirulina, chlorella, bee products, raw honey, propolis, gelatinized maca, mushrooms (reishi, chaga, cordyseps, maitake, shitake), wheatgrass juice, sunflower sprouts, pea sprouts.

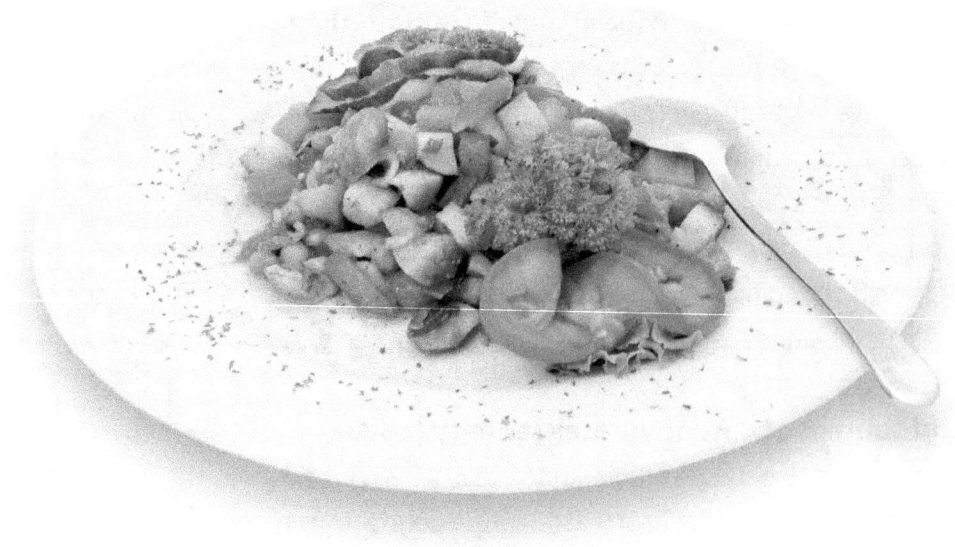

Fruit: Any seasonal organic fruit, including apples, bananas, pear, grapes

Nuts:
Almonds, walnuts, cashews

Veggies: Any seasonal and organic, including carrots, cucumbers, celery, broccoli, cauliflower, edamame

Other:
Rice cakes
Whole grain tortilla chips

Healthy add ons:
Hummus
Nut butter (almond, sunflower, organic peanut)
Avocado

Nutrition and Meal Bars:
Beware! Many on-the-go nutrition bars are loaded with sugar and chemicals. They are really not much better than candy bars. However, there are a few good ones on the market that I like.

Companies with plant-based bars that I like:
myVega.com
22days.com
Gomarco.com

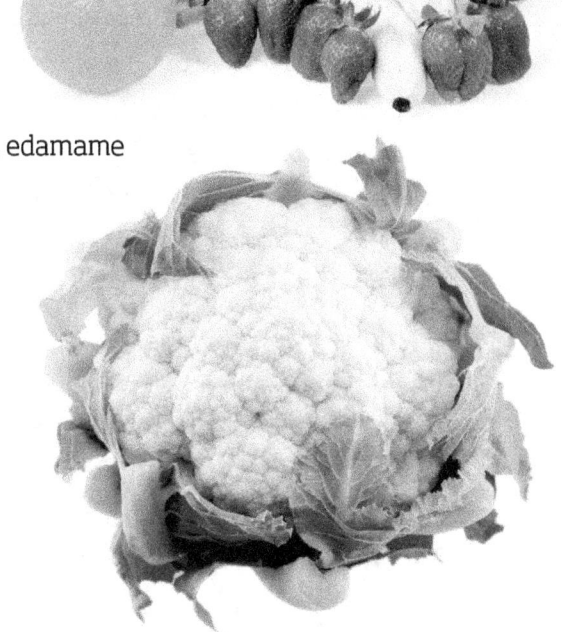

As a way of tuning into your body and listening to its messages, avoid eating the following food items for 10 days, then try reintroducing them back into your diet one day at a time and note how you feel, both right after eating and again two hours later. Take note of your energy level, mood, mental clarity and any physical symptoms you experience (bloating, gas, and diarrhea). **Avoid these food items for 10 days then reintroduce them one at a time and record how you feel after eating them.** The below list of food items are the usual suspects that most people are sensitive to.

Day 1: Dairy products - milk, cream, yogurt, cheese

Day 2: Soy - tofu, soy beans

Day 3: Sugar/artificial sweeteners - sucrose, high fructose corn syrup and chemical artificial sweeteners such as Splenda (sucralose), Sweet & Low (saccharin), Equal and NutraSweet (aspartame)

Day 4: Corn products - dextrose, corn meal, corn syrup, monosodium glutamate (MSG), maltodextrin

Day 5: Peanuts - Non organic peanut butter

Day 6: Chemical ingredients - artificial colors and flavoring, butylate hydroxyanisole (BHA) and butylated hydroxyuene (BHT), sodium nitrate and nitrite, partially hydrogenated oils (trans-fats)

Day 7: Gluten - wheat products, including wheat bread, bagels, beer, cookies, cakes, baked goods, crackers, pasta, pizza, pretzels

You may discover from this exercise that you are unusually sensitive to certain foods. A food sensitivity or allergy may be your body's way of telling you to start eating foods more appropriate for your current life goals. Avoid all foods that you find you're sensitive to.

What I ate:	How I felt right after eating:	Two hours later:
Day 1		
Day 2		
Day 3		
Day 4		
Day 5		
Day 6		
Day 7		

Determine How Many Calories to Consume

Estimating how many calories you should be consuming is based on your height, weight, age, and activity level. Basal metabolic rate or (BMR) is the amount of calories your body burns at rest, also known as your metabolism. Your BMR usually comprises as much as 65% of your total calories burned. Use the following formula to calculate your BMR or use an online BMR calculator.

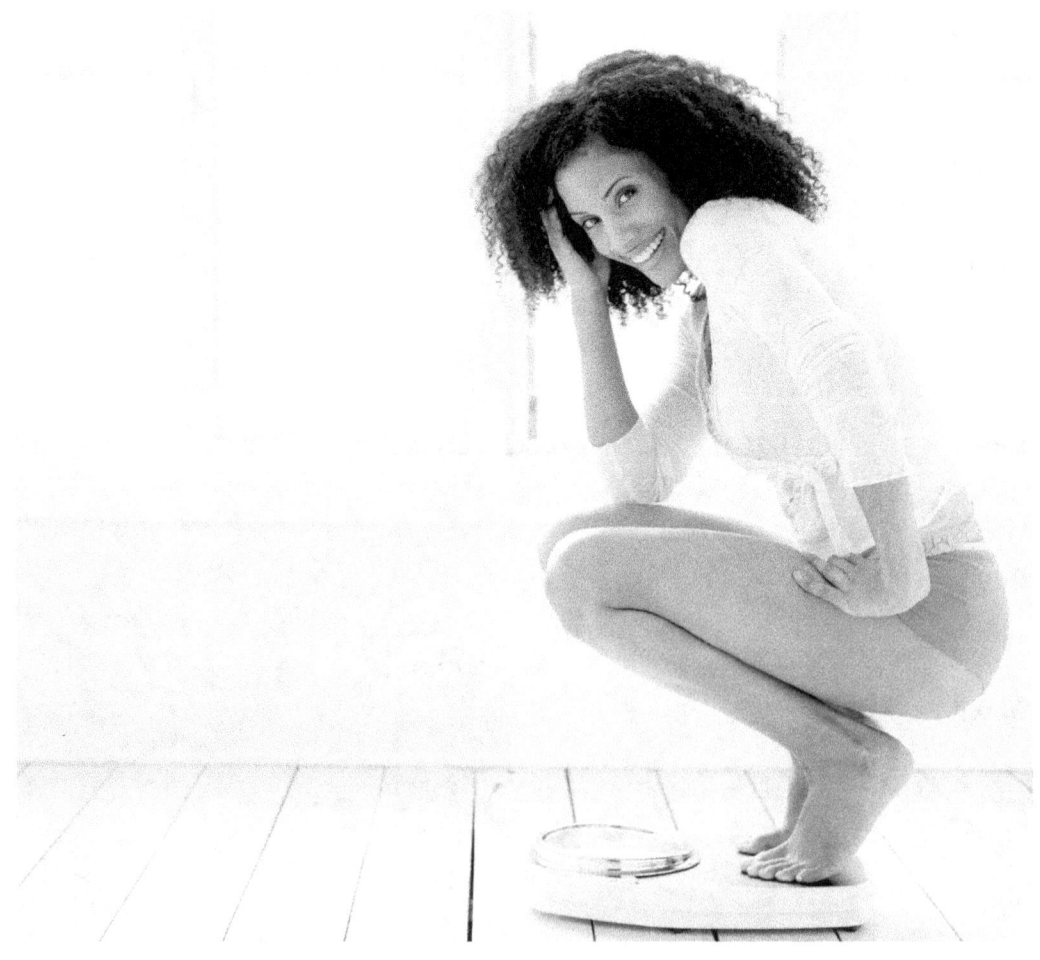

Harris-Benedict Principle:

Men	BMR = 88.362 + (13.397 x weight in kg) + (4.799 x height in cm) - (5.677 x age in years)
Women	BMR = 447.593 + (9.247 x weight in kg) + (3.098 x height in cm) - (4.330 x age in years)

Activity level

Little to no exercise	Daily kilocalories needed = BMR x 1.2
Light exercise (1-3 days per week)	Daily kilocalories needed = BMR x 1.375
Moderate exercise (3-5 days per week)	Daily kilocalories needed = BMR x 1.55
Heavy exercise (6-7 days per week)	Daily kilocalories needed = BMR x 1.725
Very heavy exercise (twice per day, extra heavy workouts)	Daily kilocalories needed = BMR x 1.9

*Your answer is the recommended daily kilocalories intake to maintain your current weight

To lose weight you'll need to intake less than your answer. 3,500 calories equals a lb of fat. So if you want to lose a lb of fat per week you'll need to go into a daily caloric defect of 500 calories per day.

Caloric Tracker Worksheet

Record the amount of calories you consume for one week.

Day	Breakfast	Lunch	Dinner	Snack	Calories
Monday					
Tuesday					
Wednesday					
Thursday					
Friday					
Saturday					
Sunday					

Note: There are many great calorie tracker applications for smart phones that make tracking calories a breeze.

These are my 3 favorites:
1. My fitness pal
2. Lose it
3. Cron-o-Meter

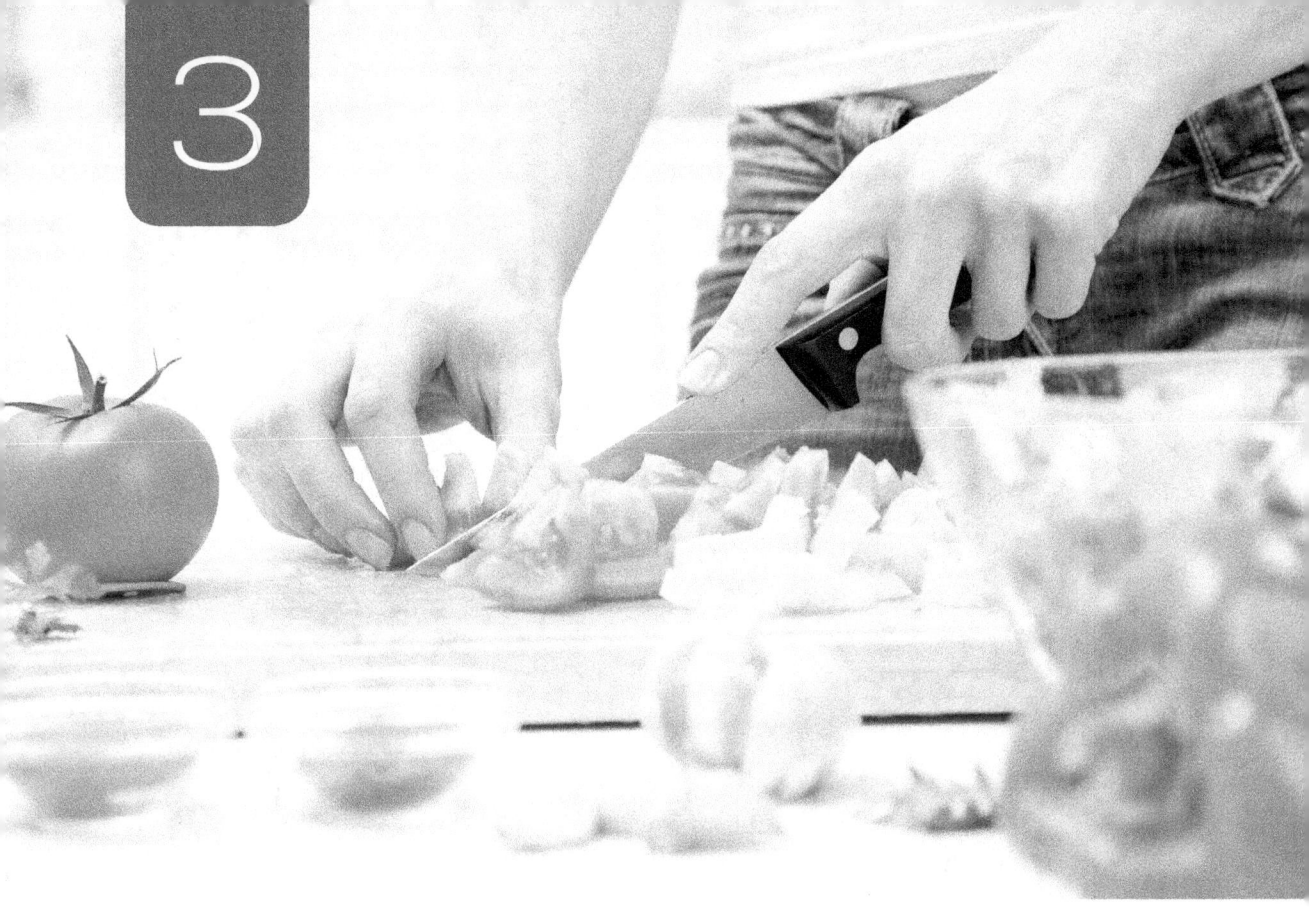

SIMPLE & EFFECTIVE STRATEGIES & TECHNIQUES

✔ Meal Planning and Preparation
✔ Creating and Implementing
Healthy Meal Options
✔ Understanding Health Food Labels
✔ Healthy Cooking Simplified

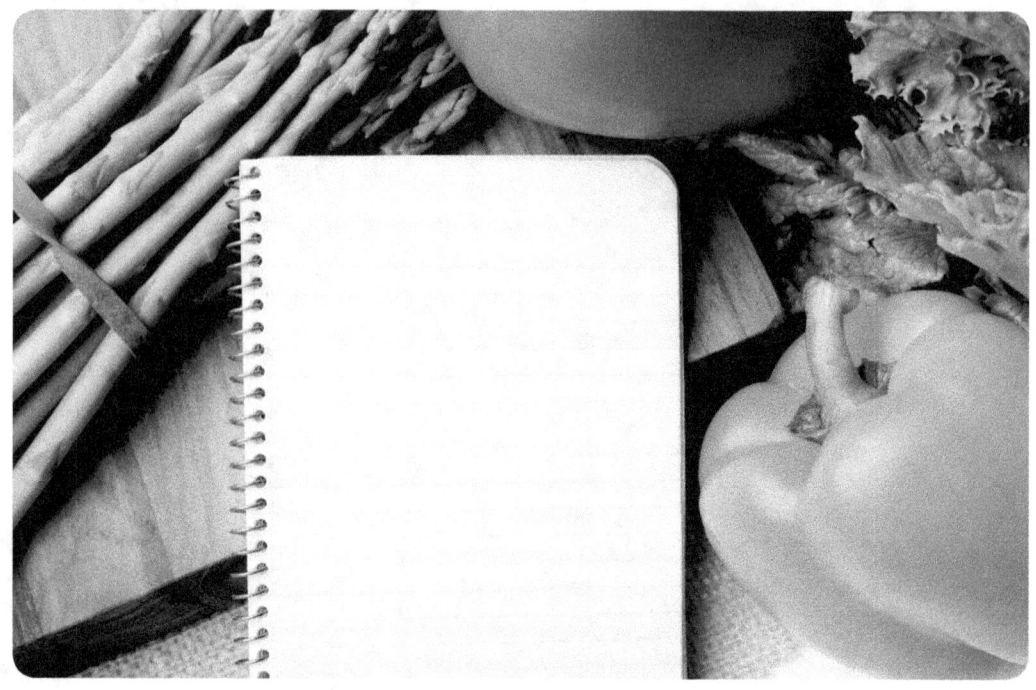

MEAL PLANNING

Meal planning is simply taking the time to plan what and when you're going to eat. This is essential to eating healthy in the 21st century especially because we all live such fast paced lives. The easiest way to start the process of meal planning is to choose a day and time, and schedule it just like you would anything else that's important in your life.

This is really a simple strategy, but is often overlooked. By planning what and when you're going to eat, you'll have healthy meals ready to go when you are, rather than being unprepared and eating whatever is around or ordering something unhealthy.

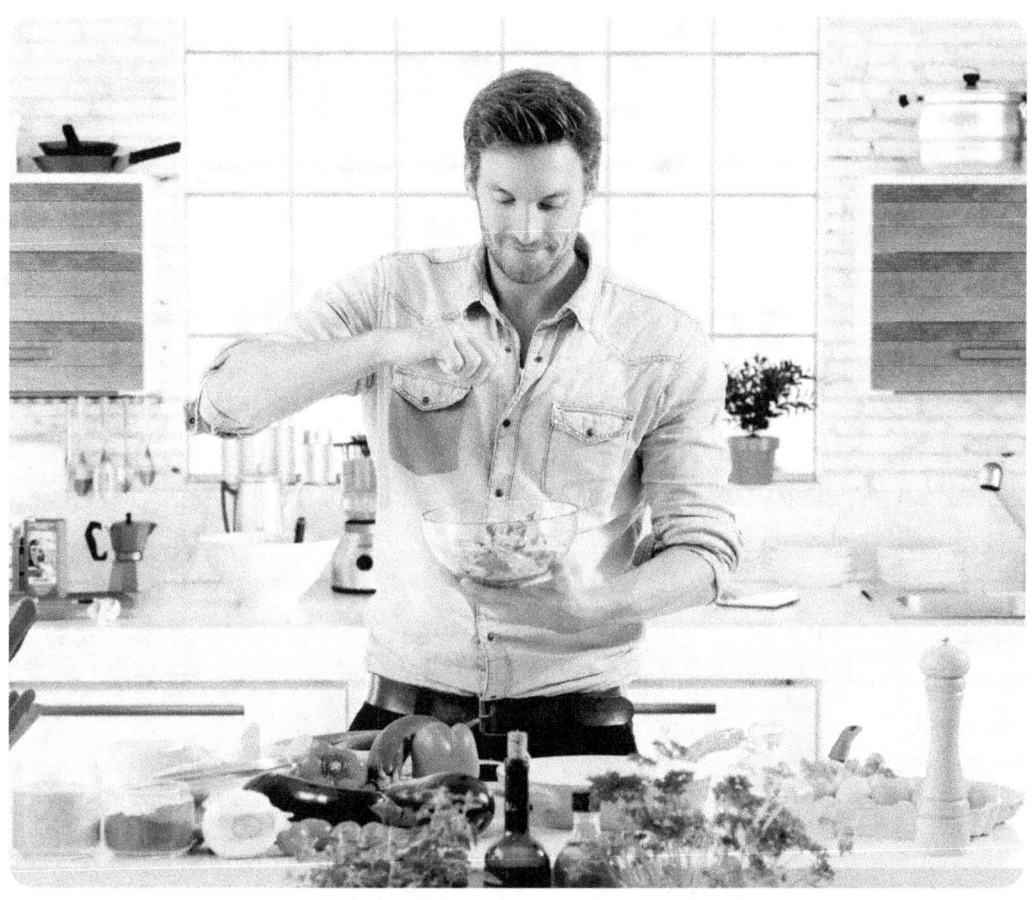

MEAL PREPARATION

After scheduling the process of meal planning, the next step is to figure out when you're going to prepare and cook your meals. A simple yet effective strategy here is to cook once and eat twice, three or even four times. By this, I mean making large quantities of healthy food such as soups or grain dishes and eating them throughout the week. You can even freeze extra portions to quickly and easily heat up later to save precious time.

CHOOSING MEAL OPTIONS

Having several healthy meal and snack options for breakfast, lunch and dinner takes the guesswork out of food shopping and meal planning. Meal options should be fast and simple to prepare and nutrient dense. This will allow you to say goodbye to fast food–and hello to healthy food, fast.

Use the meal planning and preparation worksheet [pg 117] to help you get started on choosing new healthy meal options to incorporate in your new healthy lifestyle.

Generally, people buy and eat the same food week in and week out. Humans like routine because it takes less thought energy when we're on autopilot. However, it's time to jump into the pilot seat and take control of what foods and meals you eat.

Most people rotate between 3-5 meal options for breakfast, lunch and dinner and usually these options aren't the healthiest choices, but choices that somehow became part of their routine.

I'm going to ask you to break that routine and choose 3 new nutrient dense meal options you'll enjoy and start rotating through these healthier versions of your maybe not so healthy "normal" meal choices. By having just 3 healthier meal options for breakfast, lunch and dinner you'll be well on your way to experiencing more energy, mental focus and your ideal body.

Standard 21st Century Breakfast

1. No breakfast (most people don't eat breakfast)
2. Milk with processed cereal
3. Coffee with a bagel and cream cheese
4. Doughnuts
5. Eggs and bacon/sausage fast food sandwich
6. Pancakes/waffles

Nutrient-Enhanced Healthy Eating in the 21st Century Breakfast

1. Always eat a nutrient dense breakfast
2. Steel cut oats topped with mixed organic fruit and small handful of walnuts and raw honey
3. Healthy superfood breakfast smoothie
4. A slice of sprouted grain bread with 1 tsp almond butter spread on top
5. 2-3 whole organic eggs fried in a healthy fat
6. Organic quinoa pilaf topped with organic raspberries and blueberries

Lunch/Dinner Example:

Standard 21st Century Lunch/Dinner

1. Hamburger and french fries
2. Pizza
3. White pasta and creamy alfredo sauce
4. Fried chicken or chicken wings with macaroni and cheese
5. Lunch meat sandwich and bag of chips
6. Grilled steak and mashed potatoes

Nutrient-Enhanced Healthy Eating in the 21st Century Lunch/Dinner

1. Bison burger or veggie burger on a whole grain bun and a side of steamed vegetables
2. Vegetable chili, legume soup varieties with a large salad
3. Whole grain or bean pasta with organic tomato
4. Grilled organic chicken or turkey
5. Vegetable wrap and fruit
6. Grilled wild-caught fish with a large mixed greens salad

Standard 21st Century Snacks

1. Potato chips
2. Cookies, brownies and cakes
3. Pretzels
4. Ice-cream
5. Candy bars

Nutrient-Enhanced Healthy Eating in the 21st Century Snacks

1. Any type of organic fruit
2. Handful of nuts (almond, walnut, cashew)
3. Rice cakes with almond butter on top
4. Hummus with sliced vegetables
5. Healthy snack bars (whole foods based, low in sugar selections)

As you can see from the above examples, it's easy to substitute healthier meal options for your favorite not so healthy meals options and snacks. All it takes is a little know-how, preparation and the willingness and desire to make a change. Remember, it's **small changes that yield lasting results.** Continue reading for more details on shifting to healthier meal options...

Breakfast:

Breakfast is the most important meal of the day. Breakfast is so important because your body has literally been "fasting" all night. Break-fast is breaking the nightly fast that has taken place and your body is ready for some nutrient dense clean food. Don't skip breakfast! It also helps keep your blood sugar balanced, which is very important for optimal energy. Even before breakfast, remember to drink a full glass of water with lemon upon waking. Keep a glass by your bed to remind you. This will not only keep you hydrated, but will prepare the digestive system to wake up. Here are some simple and easy balanced breakfast ideas that include complex carbohydrates, protein and good fats.

Quick Easy Favorites:

Option 1

½ cup steel cut oatmeal topped with mixed organic fruit and small handful of walnuts and raw honey.

Option 2

2-3 whole fried organic eggs with a piece of sprouted grain bread with 1 tsp almond butter spread on top.

Option 3

Healthy breakfast smoothie: ½ cup hemp or almond milk, handful of organic frozen fruit, 1 scoop plant-based protein powder.

Breakfast Staples:

- Organic eggs
- Almond butter
- Unsweetened almond, hemp or oat milk
- Sprouted grain toast
- Organic fruit: banana, apple, orange, mixed berries, pear, melon
- Plant-based protein powder
- Organic steel cut oatmeal
- Organic quinoa pilaf topped with organic raspberries and blueberries

Lunch & Dinner:

I grouped lunch and dinner together because in most cases and for most meal ideas and people, they are interchangeable. If you are following my guidelines, then you are eating smaller portions including healthy snacks. However, lunch should be your largest meal of the day. The simple thing to remember for both lunch and dinner is to eat clean, lean and lots of green.

Quick Easy Favorites:

Option 1

Grilled organic chicken, turkey or wild fish with a large mixed greens salad topped with olive oil and lemon dressing. Organic apple for dessert.

* You can put the above meal into a sprouted grain wrap for variety. Just use less lean protein to counter the added calories from the wrap if you're watching your caloric intake.

Option 2

Bison burger with whole wheat bun and a side of quinoa and steamed asparagus.

Option 3

Lentil soup with a piece of sprouted grain bread and a small side salad of mixed greens. A grapefruit for dessert.

Staples:

- Any lean, responsibly grown protein source such as, organic chicken, turkey, buffalo, wild caught fish
- Any type of green vegetable
- Mixed greens, spinach, mache, spring mix
- Any type of bean. My favorite is lentils because they are packed with protein and are quick and easy to make.

Snack Options:

Snacks are super important to a balanced diet especially if you live a busy, on the go, fast-pace lifestyle. Unfortunately, most snacks available at the grocery store are super processed and loaded with trans-fat and preservatives. When snacking, it's important to think in terms of nutrient density vs processed. Going for nutrient dense food will not only make you feel full longer, but will give you more energy to fuel your day.

Favorite Snack Option Ideas:

Option 1

Any type of organic fruit. When and where possible buy organic, what's in-season and grown locally. This ensures optimal nutrient density.

Apples, bananas, peaches, pears, plums, grapes, grapefruits, orange or a healthy clean plant-based protein smoothie (see smoothie ideas in recipe section).

*My favorites are bananas and apples because they are easy to carry and loaded with fiber and nutrients.

Option 2

Nuts: walnuts, almonds, cashews - whole or made into nut butters. Nuts are high in good essential fats so eat them in moderation. A small handful should do the trick. Seeds: pumpkin seeds, sunflower seeds, flaxseeds, chia seeds. These seeds are loaded with essential fats and nutrients.

Option 3

Beans: Hummus on top of sprouted whole grain toast, baby carrots or rice cakes. Steamed edamame or edamame beans.

Note: There are some good snack bars on the market but even more bad ones. Use this criteria when buying them.

- The less ingredients the better
- Shoot for under 10 grams of sugar per serving
- A minimally processed (made with whole foods)

HEALTHY COOKING SIMPLIFIED

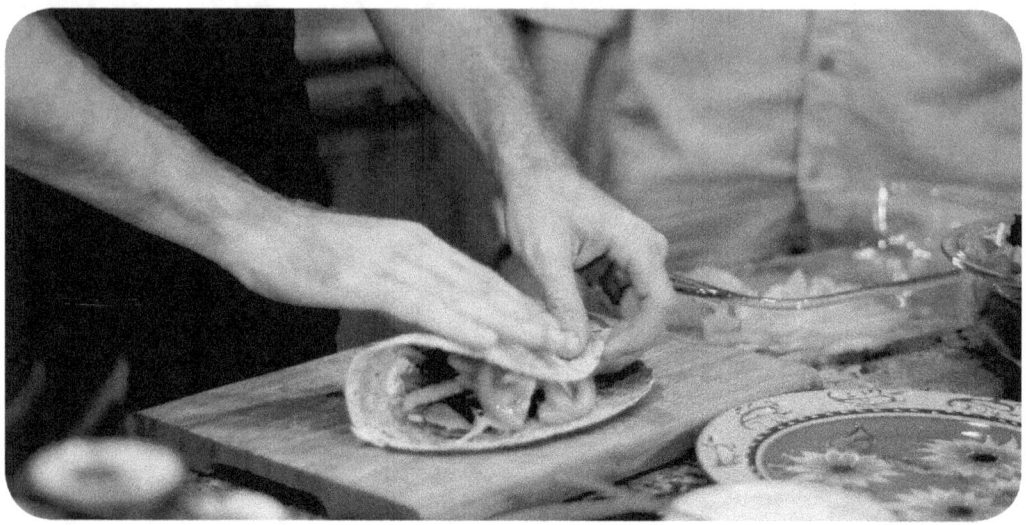

When you're busy, cooking may seem inconvenient and intimidating, especially if you're new to it. However, it's easy if you start simple and learn to cook and prepare a few quick and healthy meals. Over time, you'll learn which simple healthy meal options you like best and learn to have those ingredients on hand for fast and tasty meal creations. I know it can be challenging to eat well when you're constantly on the go, but you can save time without sacrificing your health by following these simple suggestions for easy-prep meal options.

Suggestion #1: Make it a wrap.
You can find countless combinations of lean protein, veggies and healthy sauces that taste great together when rolled into a wrap. Wraps are also a simple way to use up leftovers. For example, if you are rushing to fix a quick meal, take leftovers like vegetable bison chili, curry, or stir-fry and place a half-cup in a whole or sprouted grain tortilla. Add organic green onions, crunchy peppers, or other crisp veggies, then roll it closed and serve.

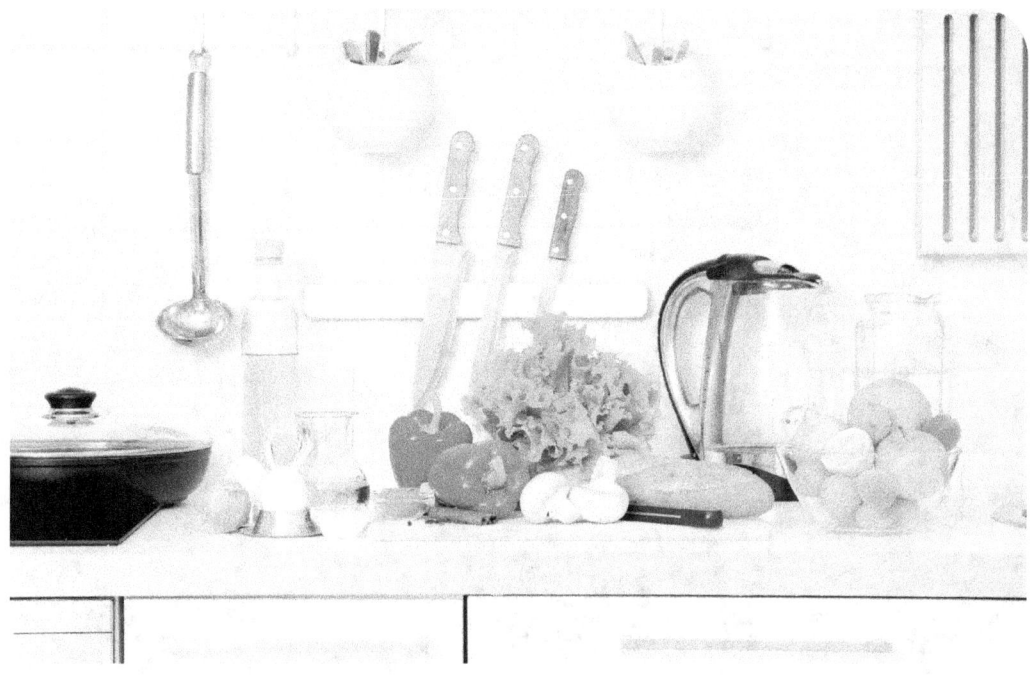

Suggestion #2: Keep it simple with your stovetop.

You can create nearly infinite stove top meals with six tools or less: a whisk, spatula, spoon, sharp knife, cutting board, and cast iron or ceramic frying pan.

Here are some stovetop staples: pan-fried wild-caught fish, organic chicken breasts, or bison burgers. Be sure to use coconut oil or grapeseed oil when pan-frying.

- Toasted veggie sandwiches
- Scrambled eggs or omelets
- Vegetable quesadillas made with whole grain wraps
- Stir-fries

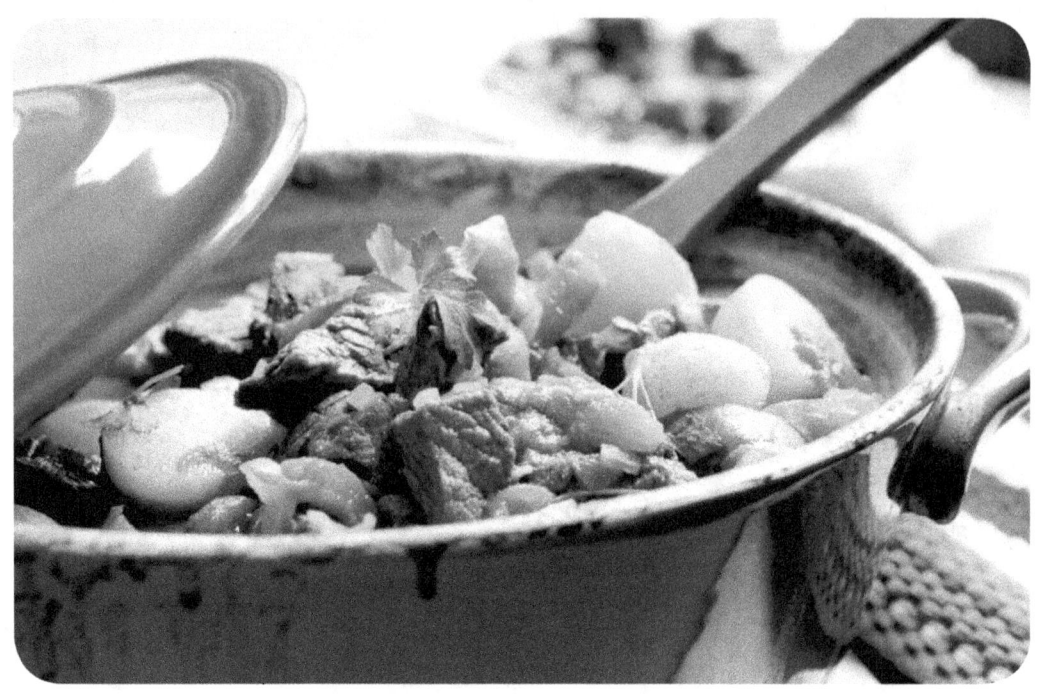

Suggestion #3: Use a crockpot for cooking.

For delicious dinners on busy weeknights, invest in a crockpot or slow cooker. Many slow-cooked recipes call for just a few simple steps and healthy affordable ingredients.

Consider this simple recipe for chicken: Rinse five or six organic chicken thighs in water and place them in your slow cooker along with a full jar of your favorite and healthy pasta sauce. Cook on low for eight hours (or set a timer and cook on high for four hours). You'll likely arrive home from work to an appetizing aroma. Next, whip up your favorite bean or whole grain pasta and top with your slow-cooked chicken and sauce.

Suggestion #4: Use healthy sauces.

A squirt of lemon juice or splash of low-sodium soy sauce may be all it takes to transform your next batch of soup, salad or stir-fry. Bottled sauces, marinades and dressings are great for turning simple staples into delicious meals. Be sure to buy products that are low in salt, sugar, and trans and saturated fat. Many of them are still full of flavor. Buy organic sauces where and when possible.

Examples:

- Lemon or lime juice
- Hot sauces
- Tomato sauce
- Soy or teriyaki sauce
- Salad dressing

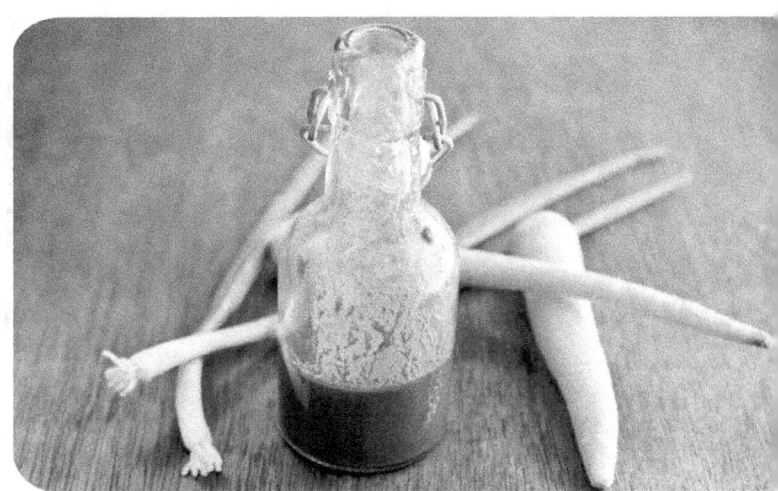

Suggestion #5: Create with convenience foods.

Keep convenience food on hand for your busiest moments. Read the labels and buy products that are low in salt, sugar, trans and saturated fat. You can mix and match them for different meal options.

For example, in moments of haste, try combining a serving of low-sodium vegetable stock with a half-cup of frozen organic veggies (such as broccoli, carrots, peas, and corn), a dash of your favorite herbs and spices. Heat it up and you'll have a hearty, flavorful, veggie-filled soup to enjoy. Another option is to top a bowl of bagged salad mix with a half-can of wild tuna. Add a spoonful of healthy salad dressing, then sprinkle with dried fruit, nuts, or your favorite veggies, and enjoy.

HEALTHY COOKING SIMPLIFIED
RECIPES

Note: Avoid canned ingredients and use 'organic' whenever possible. See page 31.

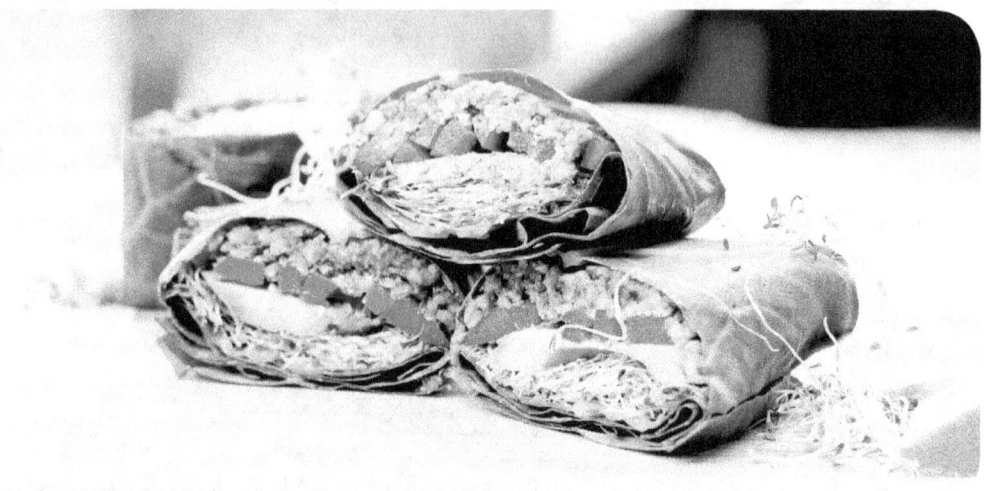

Wrap Recipes:

Southwest Bean Wrap

Ingredients:

1 whole wheat or sprouted tortilla wrap

3-4 tablespoons of southwestern hummus

2 tablespoons corn

2 tablespoons black beans

1 tablespoon diced tomato

2 tablespoons diced avocado

1 cup shredded lettuce

Directions:

Spread hummus over wrap. Layer the rest of ingredients on top of hummus. Wrap it up and enjoy!

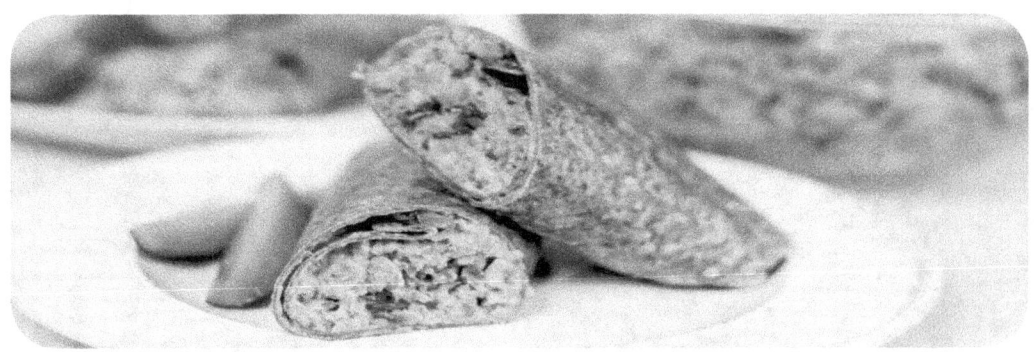

Sonia's Veggie Wrap

Ingredients:
1 sprouted whole grain wrap
¼ cup hummus
¼ cup cooked quinoa
¼ cup sliced cherry tomatoes
½ cup shredded carrots
¼ cup sliced red and green peppers
½ avocado
½ cup spring mix lettuce
1 teaspoon olive oil
pinch of sea salt

Directions:
Spread hummus on tortilla. Place quinoa, tomatoes, carrots, avocado, peppers and lettuce in tortilla. Drizzle olive oil on top and add a pinch of sea salt. Roll and enjoy!

Asian Chicken Wrap

Ingredients:
1 sprouted whole grain wrap
1 chicken breast, cooked and sliced
1/2 cup romaine lettuce
¼ teaspoon tamari sauce
¼ teaspoon teriyaki sauce
1/3 cup shredded carrots

Directions:
Combine sauces and heat until boiling. Lower heat. Simmer sauce until thickened. Place chicken slices in a bowl. Add the sauce. Mix until chicken is coated. Prepare wrap. Place romaine lettuce, chicken, and carrots in the center of the tortilla. Roll and enjoy.

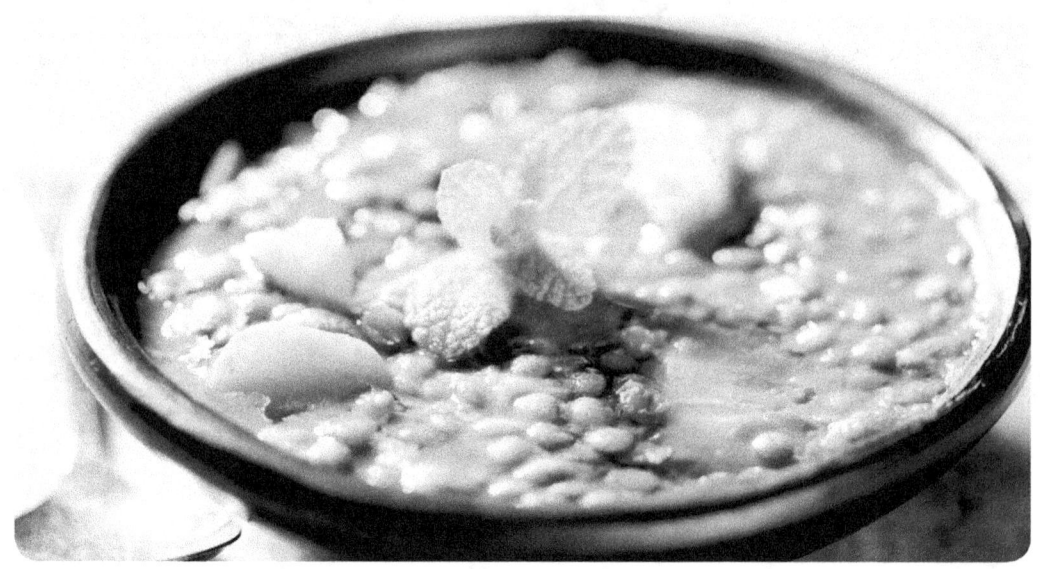

Lentil Crockpot Soup

Ingredients:

1 white onion, chopped

2 carrots, cut on the bias or rolled cut

1 pound mushrooms

½ cup dried green lentils

16 ounces black beans, drain if canned

2 cups diced tomatoes

1 can whole kernel corn

½ teaspoon dried basil

½ teaspoon dried oregano

½ teaspoon dried parsley

½ teaspoon salt

¼ teaspoon black pepper

⅛ teaspoon garlic powder

⅛ teaspoon onion powder

⅛ teaspoon dried thyme

⅛ teaspoon dried rosemary

32 ounces vegetable broth

Directions:

Add everything to the crock pot and stir.

Cook on low 8 to 10 hours or on high 4 to 5 hours.

Chicken, Sweet Potato, Quinoa Crockpot Soup

Ingredients:

1 and 1/2 pounds boneless skinless chicken breasts

1 cup quinoa (I use a black bean quinoa package)

2 large sweet potatoes (1 pound or 3-1/2 cups)

15.25 ounces black beans

½ cup diced tomatoes

1 teaspoon minced garlic

1 teaspoon chili power

5 cups chicken broth

Optional: fresh parsley

Directions:

Put chicken breasts, quinoa, and chopped sweet potatoes into the crock pot. Add black beans, diced tomatoes, minced garlic, chili powder, and chicken broth. Cook on high for 3-5 hours. Using two forks, shred the chicken and stir all the ingredients together. Add salt and pepper, and fresh parsley if desired.

Tortilla Crockpot Soup

Ingredients:
14.5 ounces diced tomatoes

1 can red enchilada sauce

14-16 ounces black beans, drained & rinsed if canned

1 medium onion, chopped

¼ cup chopped green chile peppers

2 cloves garlic, minced

1 package frozen corn (about 14 ounces)

29 ounces vegetable broth

1 teaspoon cumin

1 teaspoon chili powder

1 teaspoon sea salt

1/4 teaspoon pepper

1 bay leaf

2 whole wheat tortillas

Directions:
Place tomatoes, enchilada sauce, black beans, onion, green chiles, corn and garlic into pot. Pour in vegetable broth, and add cumin, chili powder, salt, pepper, and bay leaf. Cover and cook on low setting for 6 to 8 hours or on high setting for 3 to 4 hours.

Preheat oven to 400 degrees. Cut tortillas into strips using a pizza cutter, then spread on a baking sheet. Add a pinch of seasoning of choice or sea salt.

Bake in preheated oven until crisp, about 10 to 15 minutes. Top with avocado, green onions and sprinkle tortilla strips on top. Serve and enjoy!

Green Goodness Salad Dressing

Ingredients:

(Makes 1 cup)
1/2 avocado, skin removed and pitted
2 tablespoons lemon juice
1 clove garlic, minced
1/4 cup fresh parsley
2 scallions
1 teaspoon sesame oil
1/4 teaspoon sea salt
2 dates, soaked in hot water for 2 minutes
1/2 teaspoon ginger, peeled and grated
3/4 cup water

Directions:

Place all ingredients into blender and blend until smooth and creamy. Enjoy.

Simple Lemon Dressing/ Sauce

Ingredients:

⅓ cup fresh squeezed lemon juice
¼ cup + 3 tablespoons olive oil
¼ cup coconut vinegar (or white wine vinegar)
3 tablespoons raw honey
¼ teaspoon sea salt
¼ teaspoon black pepper

Directions:

Add all ingredients to a jar or bowl. Shake or mix together until fully combined.

Sesame Ginger Miso Sauce

1 tablespoon sesame seeds

1.5 tablespoons tamari sauce

2 tablespoons olive oil

4 tablespoons honey

3 tablespoons roasted sesame oil

4 tablespoons rice vinegar

Ingredients:

2" peeled fresh ginger

3 tablespoons miso

Juice of one lime or lemon

Directions:

Add all ingredients to a food processor or blender and blend until smooth. Use on top of a salad or chicken dish.

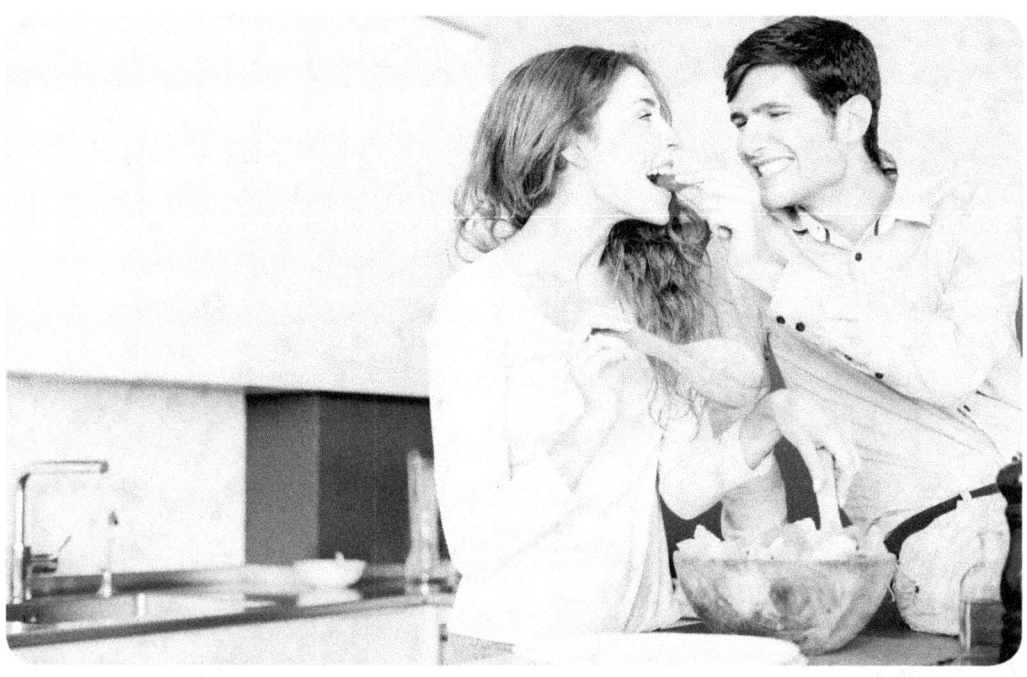

Healthy Convenience Food Ideas

Fast Soup

Ingredients:

1 can low sodium soup

1 cup frozen mixed vegetables

¼ cup water

Directions:

Combine. Heat. Eat

Swift Salad

Ingredients:

Greens of your choice - 3 cups

2 teaspoons dressing of your choice

¼ cup dried nuts (almonds and walnuts)

¼ cup pumpkin seeds

½ cup wild tuna

Directions:

Combine. Eat.

THE ART OF UNDERSTANDING "HEALTHY" FOOD LABELS

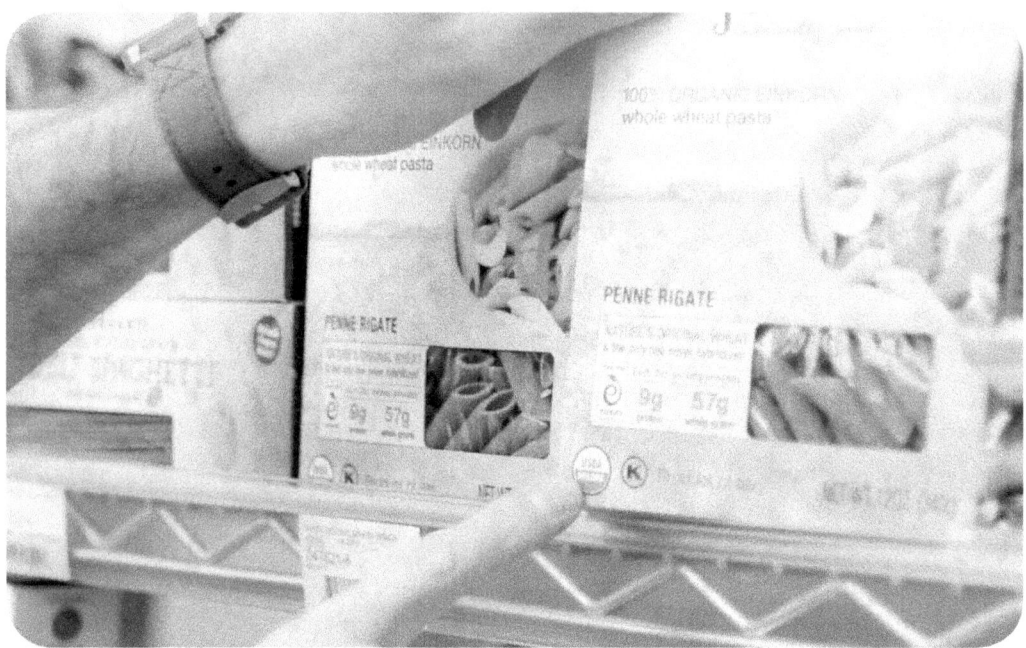

Unfortunately, it's not just the industrial food producers that have tricky labeling terms when it comes to buying food. Healthy food marketers also use labeling to draw health conscious consumers to their products. Below are some labeling terms explained, so you can get the most bang for your buck when it comes to buying truly healthy food.

"No hormones added or administered": This label means that no hormones have been used over the animal's lifetime. Unfortunately, there is no organization standing behind this claim, other than the company producing the products. Eighty percent of all U.S. feedlot cattle are injected with synthetic hormones. Although you will see this label used for poultry and pork, it is all marketing because poultry and pork are federally prohibited from being injected with hormones.

"Raised without antibiotics": This label means that through the animal's lifetime, no antibiotics were given or administered. Since there is no third party verification, this claim is only somewhat meaningful.

"Kosher": This label only means that the products have been prepared under a rabbi's supervision. It doesn't include any environmental, health or welfare standards.

"Humane": There is no legal or regulatory definition of this claim. Different companies use this claim for different meanings.

"Certified Humane": Means that a third party has verified and confirmed that the producers adhered to strict animal welfare guidelines. (So if you care about how the animal was treated while it was alive, look for this labeling term.)

"Certified Organic": Only food producers who adhere to strict United States Department of Agriculture (USDA) standards can have this organic label. Organic livestock is not given antibiotics or growth hormones, are fed only organically produced feed and must have access to a pasture.

"Grass-fed": This label is meant to mean that the animal was only fed one hundred percent grass during its lifetime. However, there is no third party verification and some unethical producers have been known to feed their animals grain, inject hormones and antibiotics and still use the label. To be safe, look for the following meaningful labels: American Grassfed Association, Grassfed USDA Process Verified, Food Alliance Grassfed, Animal Welfare Approved, Demeter Biodynamic and GAP Step 5+, 5 and 4.

"Free Range": This label means that the animals may have been allowed outside access which could only be a small open door or window in a crowded barn. There is no third party verification for this claim. The producer or manufacturer decides whether to use the claim and is not free from its own self-interest.

Common General "Health Food" Labeling Terms

"All natural": This labeling term simply means that the food was minimally processed. Food companies love to use this one to sway health conscious consumers....beware!

"Fresh": Only means that the food has not been frozen (below 26 degrees F).

"No additives": A general claim that may imply a product (or packaging) has not been enhanced with the addition of natural or artificial ingredients. There is no guidance for the use of the claim "no additives" from the U.S. Food and Drug Administration (FDA) or the USDA.

Generally, the best food labels are the seals or logos indicating that an independent organization has verified that a product meets a set of meaningful and consistent standards for environmental protection and food safety. Look for '*certified*' in the label.

Eighty-five certifying agents are currently USDA-accredited and authorized to
certify operations to the USDA organic standards. Of these, forty-nine are based in
the U.S. and thirty-six are based in foreign countries. These private companies must
certify that the farm complies with the standards, often hiring a collector in the
area to send samples to a lab. Secondly, the National Organic Program (NOP), and in
Canada the CFIA, perform random sampling as well.

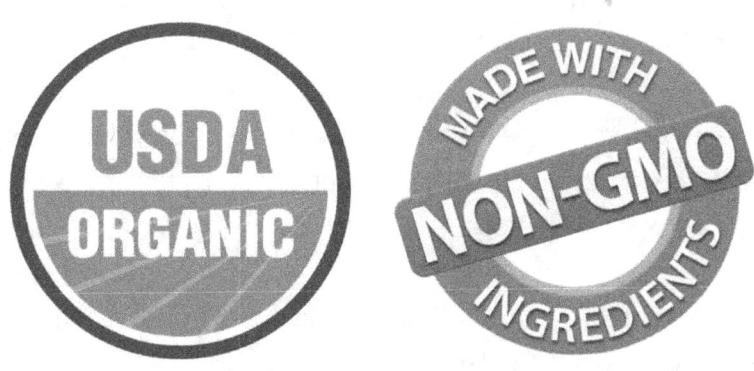

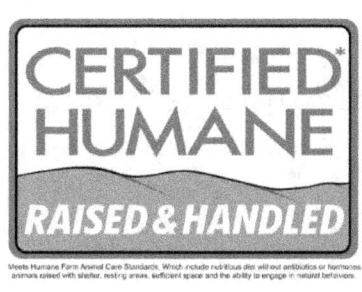

What to look for when reading a food label...

1. Check the serving size and total calories. Many food labels only show the nutritional facts for just one serving when they contain multiple servings. Be sure to look at the serving size on the package to determine how many servings you are actually eating.

2. Make calories count. Eat nutrient dense foods that are low in calories and high in nutrition. To determine if a food is nutrient dense, look at the label and compare the nutrients to the amount of calories. Processed foods are high in calories and low in nutrients.

3. Check the sugar content. Make sure added sugars (sucrose, glucose, high fructose corn syrup, corn syrup and fructose) are not one of the first ingredients and preferably not even on the label.

4. Check the fat content. Eating foods low in saturated, trans fat and cholesterol reduces the risk of heart disease.

5. Check the sodium content. Choose foods low in sodium. Salt intake is directly related to high blood pressure. The recommended daily allowance is no more than 2,400 mg or about 1 tsp. of salt a day.

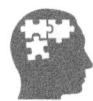

Key Concepts

1. Meal planning is simply taking the time to plan what and when you're going to eat. This is essential to eating healthy in the 21st century. Meal planning must be a priority in your life.

2. Choosing several healthy meal options for breakfast, lunch and dinner and learning to cook them takes the guesswork out of food shopping and meal preparation.

3. Learn the art of "healthy food" label reading. Even "healthy" food marketers can use tricky labeling to draw you to their products. Know what labeling terms actually mean. Review pg.103-104.

4. Know what to look for when reading a food label. Check the serving size and total calories. Make calories count. Processed foods are high in calories and low in nutrients. Check the sugar content. Check the fat content. Check the sodium content.

Action Items

✓ Take time right now to schedule when you're going to plan your meals.

✓ Choose a few new healthy meal options to try. Use the healthy recipes section for ideas.

✓ For convenience, fill large jars or glass containers with different nuts, seeds and dried superfoods to include them into your simple easy meal options.

✓ Review the health food labeling keywords [pg 102-104] so you know what to look for and what to avoid in the grocery store. Use the essential shopping list as your guide [pg 113].

CHAPTER 3:
SUPPLEMENTAL MATERIALS

Healthy Recipe Idea Section

Breakfast

Energizing Oatmeal

1/2 cup steel cut oats (1 cup cooked)

2 cups water

Sea salt to taste

Top with:

¼ cup wild blueberries (fresh or frozen)

¼ cup raspberries (fresh or frozen)

2 teaspoons crushed almonds and pumpkin

seeds

Cinnamon to taste

Note: Cooking steel cut oats takes about 30 minutes. Make a big batch and separate into individual portions to be heated up quickly on the stovetop when ready to use.

Easy Egg Sandwich

2 slices sprouted whole grain bread

3 whole eggs (fried, scrambled or poached)

Slice of tomato

Cholula hot sauce to taste

Quick Breakfast Burrito

4 egg whites

Sautéed onions and peppers

1 cup spinach

¼ cup cherry tomatoes

Whole grain tortilla

Cholula hot sauce to taste

Plant Power Smoothie

Blend...

1 cup unsweetened almond or flax milk

¼ cup frozen wild organic blueberries

¼ cup frozen organic raspberries

1 frozen banana

1 scoop plant-based protein (my favorite Vega Essential-All-in-One French Vanilla)

Add in superfoods to super charge it

1 teaspoon chia seeds

1 teaspoon gelatinized maca powder

Healthy Cereals

There are some healthy cereals available for purchase.

Shoot for one that is organic, low in sugar, high in fiber and made of whole grains.

Eat with 1 cup unsweetened almond or flax milk, and top with

1 teaspoon wild raw honey and ½ cup fresh organic berries.

Lunch & Dinner

Wonderful Wrap

Whole grain wrap

½ avocado, sliced

1 cup spinach or mixed greens

¼ cup quinoa

Sliced tomato

5 ounces sliced baked chicken or wild fish

* Wraps are simple, easy and fast to make. Experiment with filling them with different whole grains, veggies and clean/lean protein sources.

Super Salad

2 cups spinach or mix greens

½-1 cup beans (lentil, black, pinto, garbanzo and/or butterbean)

Sliced cucumbers, tomatoes, peppers, avocado

¼ cup walnuts or almonds

1 teaspoon chia or flax seeds

Dress with 1 teaspoon olive oil and ½ squeezed lemon

Baked Chicken & Veggies

6 ounce organic chicken breast

Seasoning options:

Thyme, basil, sea salt, black pepper, garlic or onion powder, cumin, paprika. Place in glass cookware and bake at 350 for 20-30 minutes until cooked. Season 1 cup asparagus, broccoli, or cauliflower and coat with 1 teaspoon olive oil. Place in pan and bake until crisp-tender.

Grill & Greens

6 ounces grilled and seasoned organic chicken, turkey or wild fish
3 cups large mixed green salad with 1 teaspoon olive oil and lemon dressing
Top with mixed nuts, feta, quinoa, tomatoes, cucumbers and peppers

Buffalo Soldier Burger

Bison meat formed into ¼ pound patties –
grilled or baked
Whole wheat bun
Sliced tomato
½ cup spinach
1 teaspoon dijon mustard

Optional Meal Sides

1/3 cup cooked quinoa

1 cup steamed asparagus

Super Soup and Salad

1 cup lentil soup
1 slice of sprouted grain bread
1 cup small side salad of mixed greens
½ a grapefruit

*Not all foods on this list will be ideal for everyone. We each have different biochemical make ups and therefore digest and assimilate foods differently. Use this list as a guide. Listen to your body to see what foods are right for your individual needs by using the Bio-Food Identifier Worksheet on page 74.

Frozen foods:
- Grass fed tenderloin
- Organic chicken and turkey breast
- Organic frozen mixed berries
- Organic frozen vegetables
- Assorted wild fish, wild fish burgers
- Organic bison burgers
- Artic Ice ice-cream substitute pints

Refrigerated foods:
- Fresh salsa (read label to look for preservatives)
- Organic hummus
- Organic unsweetened coconut, almond or flax milk
- Assorted seasonal organic vegetables and fruits
- Organic spinach, 50/50 mix, mache greens, or spring mix
- Organic eggs
- Assorted whole grain wraps or sprouted whole grain wraps
- Dark chocolate 70% cocoa or higher

Dry Storage Foods:

- Brown rice
- Quinoa high antioxidant trail mix (raisins, pumpkin seeds, almonds, walnuts, goji and acai berries, mulberries, berries, cranberries)
- Fast cooking steel cut oats
- Brown rice or quinoa pasta
- Organic pasta sauce
- Organic pesto sauce
- Assorted nuts and seeds
- Assorted beans
- Assorted lentils

Oils for Cooking:

- Coconut or grapeseed oil for high temperature cooking
- Olive oil for medium temperature cooking
- Extra virgin olive oil for raw use only

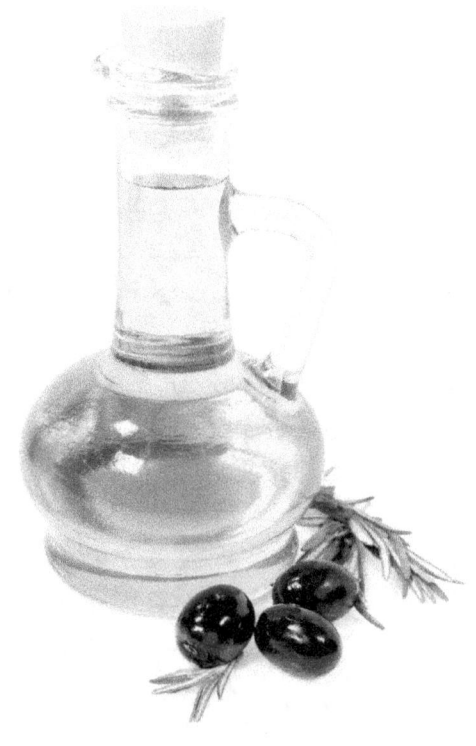

Meal Planning and Preparation Overview

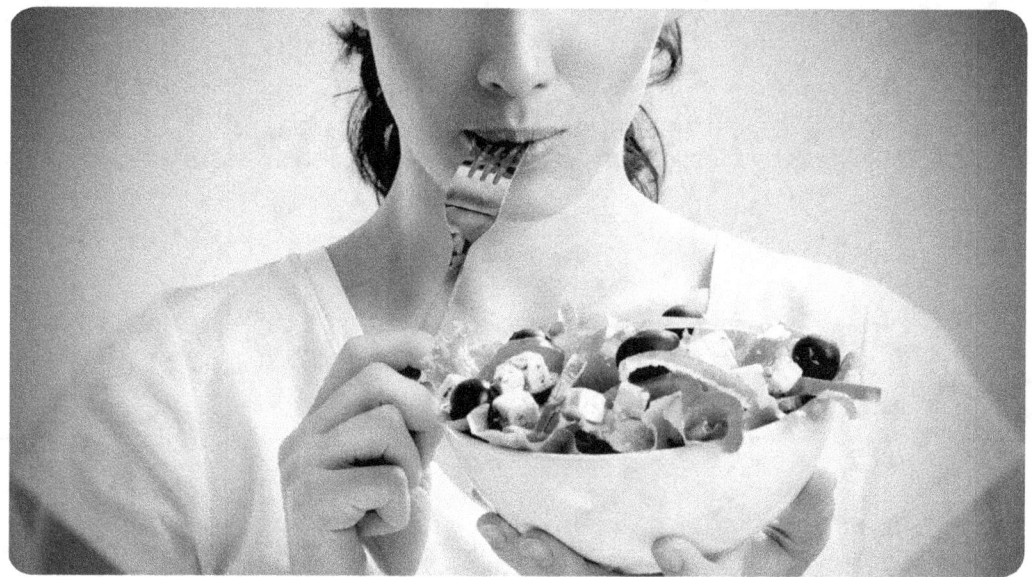

Use this guide until you're comfortable planning, shopping, cooking and preparing healthy, simple meals. Really commit to this process. It can take a little extra time in the beginning, but is well worth the pay off in the end. After a few weeks, this process will become second nature.

STEP ONE:

Plan your meals and meal times using the worksheet on page 117.
Choose 3 new healthy meal options each for breakfast, lunch and dinner.

STEP TWO:

Schedule your food shopping day and time.

STEP THREE:

Schedule meal preparation/cooking day and time.

Weekly Meal Planning and Preparation Worksheet

Monday:

Breakfast- Time	Meal option
Lunch - Time	Meal option
Dinner- Time	Meal option

Tuesday:

Breakfast- Time	Meal option
Lunch - Time	Meal option
Dinner- Time	Meal option

Wednesday:

Breakfast- Time	Meal option
Lunch - Time	Meal option
Dinner- Time	Meal option

Thursday:

Breakfast- Time	Meal option
Lunch - Time	Meal option
Dinner- Time	Meal option

Friday:

Breakfast- Time	Meal option
Lunch - Time	Meal option
Dinner- Time	Meal option

Saturday/Sunday:

Breakfast- Time	Meal option
Lunch - Time	Meal option
Dinner- Time	Meal option

Weekly Snacks:

Snacks- Time	Snack options
Snacks- Time	Snack options
Snacks- Time	Snack options

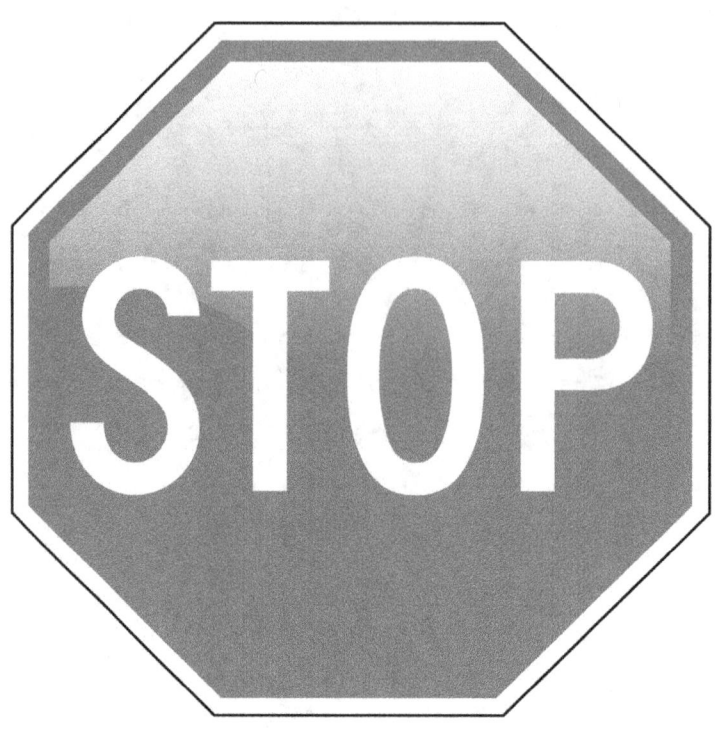

STOP!

**Did you choose 3 new healthy meal options to implement into your diet?
Did you use the meal planning worksheet to schedule your new
healthy meal options?
Did you plan your food shopping day and time?
Did you plan when you will prepare and cook your meals?**

**If you did not do any of the above recommendations, please
DO NOT continue reading until you do**
This is an **essential** part of healthy eating in the 21st century.
Take Action Now.

4

HEALTHY EATING ON THE GO

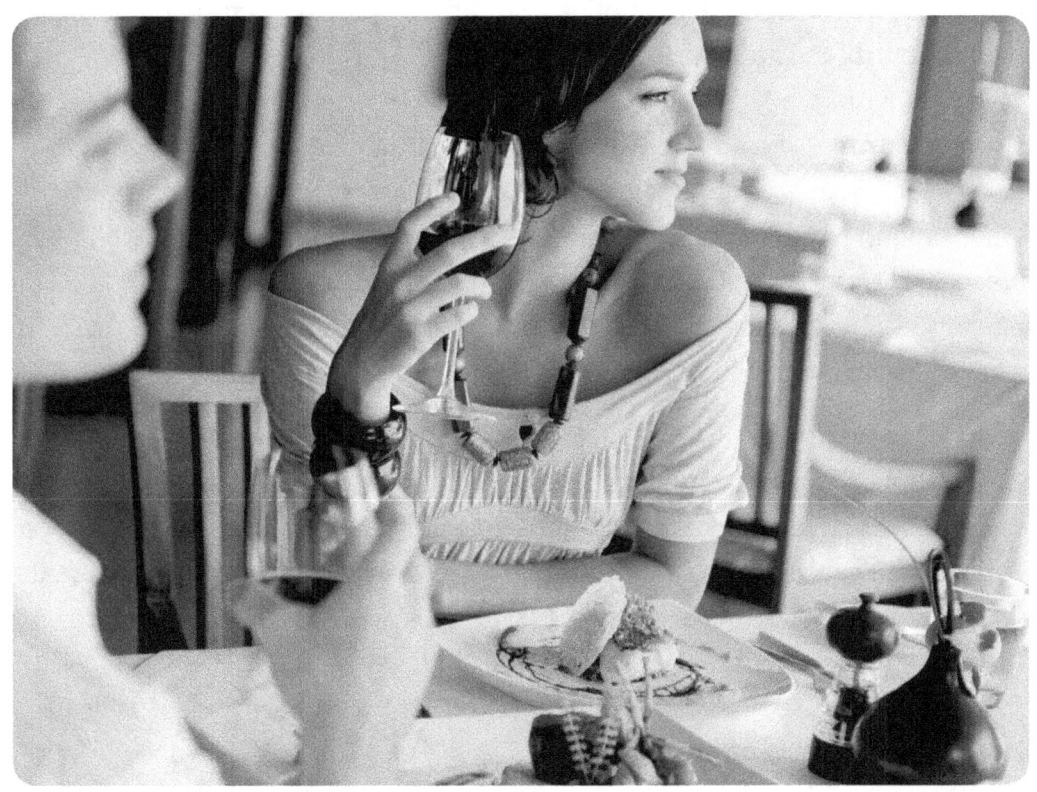

✔ Restaurants
✔ Social Events
✔ Traveling

I'd be lying if I told you that eating healthy at restaurants is easy. Unfortunately, most food and even 'clean' food is really not healthy when ordering out. There are a few things to know about eating healthier when dining at restaurants. Let's start with the obvious first. Choose a healthier restaurant over one you know will have limited healthy options. If that's not possible, consider practicing portion control and how the food is prepared.

Portion Control

Most restaurants serve huge portions of food. Either ask for a smaller portion when ordering or box up half of your meal to be eaten later. Avoid the breadbasket, ordering multiple courses and drinking alcohol with your meal. Save drinking alcohol for special occasions and drink in moderation. Following these simple recommendations will be transformative to your wasitline and health.

Food Preparation

How your meal is prepared greatly depends on how healthy it is. Even healthy food can quickly become unhealthy if it's prepared with a lot of oil, butter, salt and sugar. Let's say you go to a seafood restaurant and order baked salmon. Often restaurants will load the salmon with butter. In this case, you could order the salmon and ask for it to be prepared with minimal butter/oil. The best way to eat cooked food is either baked, broiled, grilled or steamed. **Watch out for sauces - they usually are loaded with salt, sugar and fat.** That being said, a part of being in balance is eating the things you enjoy once in a while, so don't be strict all the time.

Try This:

Next time you're dining out, instead of ordering a main course, choose to combine healthy sides to eat as a main course. If the sides are too small, just add a salad. Ask for dressing and sauces on the side (usually loaded with sugar and fat) or choose vegetable based sauces and dressings. If you know your options are going to be very limited, consider eating something healthy before you go out or eat a small portion of something on the "not-so-healthy" list.

Healthy Restaurant Finders Web Resources:

www.sustainabletable.org
www.eatwellguide.org
www.happycow.net

Traveling

Traveling can be another tricky situation for healthy eating on the go. The key here is to be prepared and have a healthy eating plan. Airport food is often very unhealthy. Try to eat before you travel so you're not stuck with limited options, and pack healthy snacks in case you get hungry along the way. If you travel often, create a *travel eating* checklist. Visit the supplemental materials on page 124 for an example. You may also find it beneficial to select a few healthy easy to carry meal/snack items and have them ready to go when you are.

Weekends

Weekends are often the toughest times to eat healthy food. For most people the weekend is a time to kick back, relax and enjoy. You worked hard all week and it's time to indulge. The trick here is to be flexible when eating for the weekends. But be smart about it. If you know you're going to be eating unhealthy at the BBQ you're attending, make sure you eat a healthy nutrient dense breakfast. Again, it's really all about finding balance. Becoming too dogmatic or strict is not balanced or healthy.

Social Events

Social events can be another challenging time to eat healthy. If you know there won't be any healthy options at the social event you're planning to attend, consider eating a healthy meal beforehand or bringing a healthy meal to the event. Obviously, use your discretion when attending social events. Being flexible and staying in balance is the key to success. Remember the 90/10 rule from pg 43. Allowing social events to fall into your 10 percent is an easy way to stay in balance without feeling deprived.

Key Concepts

1. When dining out at restaurants, use portion control. You don't have to eat everything on your plate. Save some for another meal or a snack. Request that your food is prepared with less or no oils, salts and sugars. Avoid eating fried foods; instead have your meal steamed, baked, broiled or grilled. Avoid or ask for dressings, sauces and salsa on the side.

2. When traveling or at social events, plan ahead and bring a healthy alternative or snack to prevent yourself from the temptation of eating unhealthy.

3. Don't be too strict! Eat your favorite 'not-so-healthy' foods on the weekends. Make this part of your 10 percent.

Action Item

✔ Next time you're "on-the-go" remember to try out these strategies and techniques for eating nutrient dense living foods and staying in balance.

CHAPTER 4:
SUPPLEMENTAL MATERIALS
Travel Smart to Stay Healthy

Check flight times and schedule time to eat something healthy before heading to the airport. Search for healthy food options at the airport terminal or train station ahead of time. Key is to be prepared!

Pack healthy snacks into zip lock bags for traveling:
- Fruits: banana, apple, pear, any organic easy to carry seasonal fruit works
- Nuts and seeds
- Natural meal protein bars

My Favorite Travel Healthy Eating Products:
1. Aloha's green powder packets, **www.aloha.com**
2. Navitas' natural power snack, **www.navitasnaturals.com**
3. Granola with coconut macrobar, **www.gomacro.com**
4. Apple and banana with raw almond butter, **www.artisanafoods.com**
5. 22 days protein bar, **www.22daysnutrition.com**

Healthy Eating Checklist:

☐ Check flight time(s)
☐ Schedule what and when you'll eat
☐ Prepare and pack healthy snacks

5

BRINGING IT ALL TOGETHER

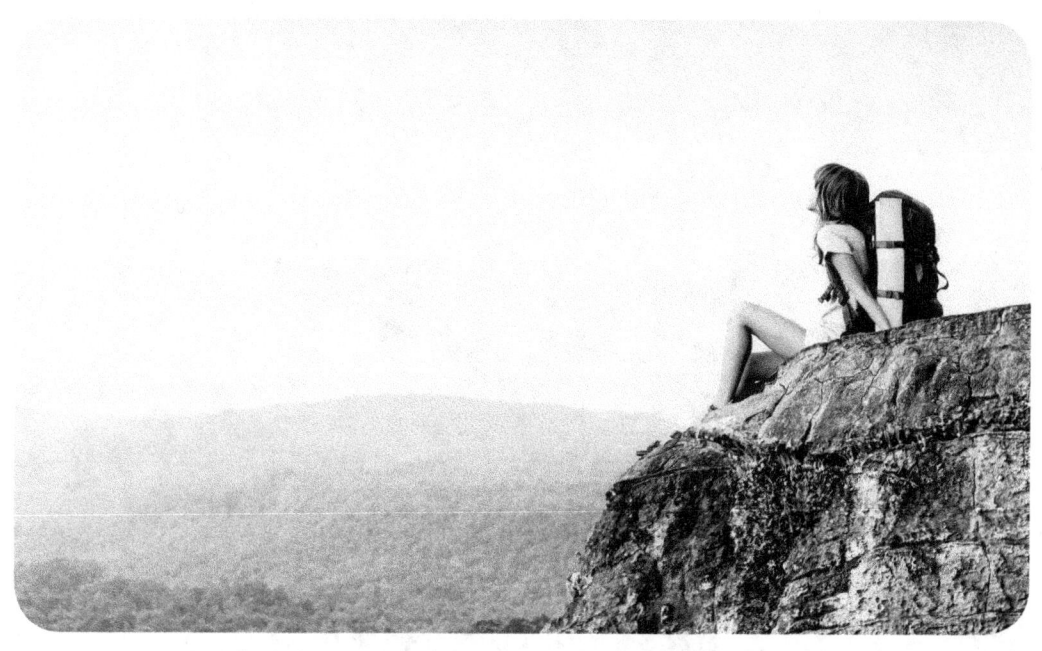

✔ Review Key Concepts
✔ Fill out Moving Forward Worksheet
✔ Congratulations

KEY CONCEPTS

Chapter 1:
WHAT NOT TO EAT
Dangers and Misinformation
in our Current Food System

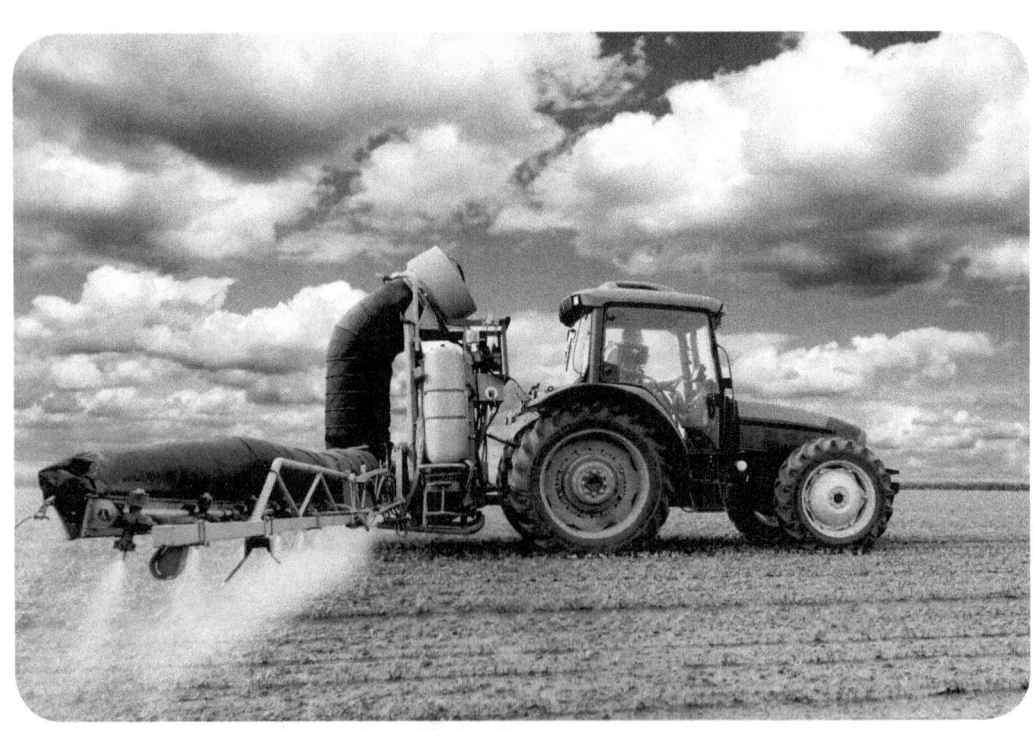

1. Our current food producing system is dangerous and not sustainable. More energy is now used to produce synthetic fertilizers than to till, cultivate and harvest all the crops in the U.S. Three billion tons of topsoil erodes from crop lands in the U.S. each year, and much is due to conventional farming practices, which ignore the health of the soil which is where our food gets its nutrients.

Unhealthy Soil = Nutrient Depleted Plants = Nutrient Depleted People = Disease.

2. We literally are what we eat. Our food goes into our stomach and is digested and absorbed into our blood which then creates our cells, tissues, organs, even our thoughts. We feel and think differently based on what we eat. The better the quality the food, the better the quality the YOU.

3. Processed artificial food products, may look and even smell like real food, but they are far from what nature intended us to eat. They are loaded with refined sugars, trans-fats and all types of other artificial chemicals to make them look and taste similar to real food, at the expense of our health. Avoid all processed artificial foods and food chemicals.

4. Conventionally grown food is food that has been exposed to pesticides, herbicides, antibiotics, growth hormones and exposed to the process of irradiation and genetic modification. This "food" negatively impacts your health and should be avoided when and where possible.

5. Ingredients and processes to avoid: GMOs; artificial flavor, color and additives; MSG; sugar, especially high fructose corn syrup and artificial sweeteners; and trans fat.

6. Gluten is found in many unhealthy processed foods and some people are highly sensitive to it. Be mindful to how you feel when you eat it.

7. If you consume dairy products, make sure you're buying them organic to avoid antibiotics and growth hormones.

8. Food manufacturers engineer addictions into their food products. To avoid being a junk food addict, avoid their engineered products.

KEY CONCEPTS

Chapter 2:
What to Eat Now: Foods that will Energize the Mind and Body

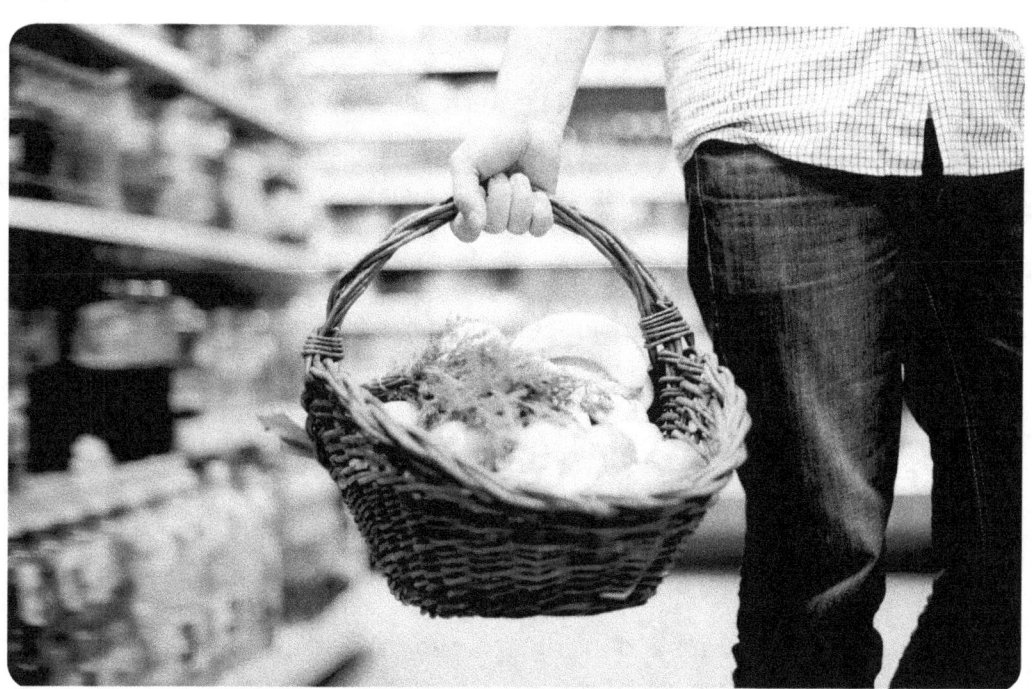

1. Eat nutrient dense, plant-based, living food that has been grown mindfully and responsibly. Buying organic food when and where possible eliminates the risks of the current dangers of our modern food production methods.

2. Go plant-based. Going plant-based simply means that your diet consist of mostly food from nutrient dense plant sources. Shoot for 70% of your total diet to be from nutrient dense plant sources.

3. Living foods are those that were once alive and still contain some of the energy (life force) that once allowed it to be. Fruits, vegetables and superfoods that are not processed are all living foods. Living food is not found in a can, bag or package.

4. Incorporate superfoods into your diet. Superfoods are the most potent, super nutrient rich foods on the planet. They have the ability to increase energy, detoxify the body, boost the immune system, lower inflammation in the body and completely nourish our bodies at the cellular level, which is where true healing takes place.

5. Eat wild-caught fish and antibiotic and hormone free animal protein sources. The better the quality of life the animal had, the better the quality the protein, thus the healthier for you.

6. Listen to your body and eat according to what it tells you. There is no one size fits all diet. Choose living, nutrient dense foods that work for you.

7. Good carbohydrates, fats and the right amount of protein are essential to looking and feeling your absolute best.

8. Calories are a measurement of energy. They are found in proteins, carbohydrates and fats. It's important to know your daily caloric needs to maintain an optimal weight.

9. An easy-to-follow rule of thumb: one-fourth of a medium-sized plate should be devoted to a starch (complex carb), another one-fourth of the plate to a lean protein (wild fish, organic poultry, beans) and the remaining half to preferably vegetables, but mostly vegetables. Fruit is best eaten in between meals for optimal digestablity.

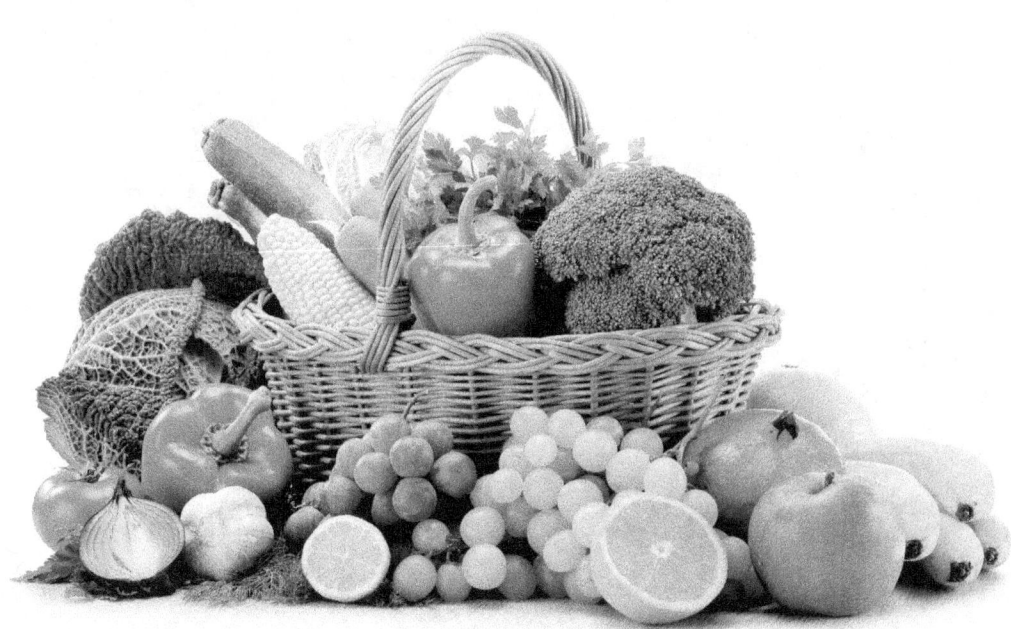

KEY CONCEPTS

Chapter 3:
Simple Effective
Strategies and Techniques

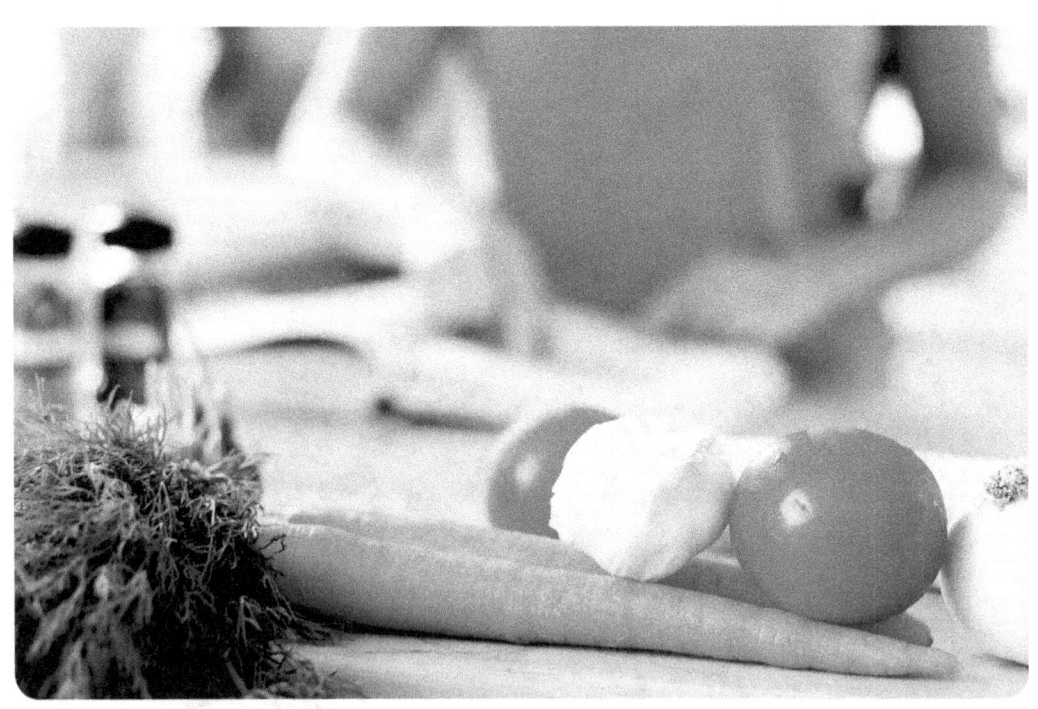

1. Meal planning is simply taking the time to plan what and when you're going to eat. This is essential to eating healthy in the 21st century. Create a habit of planning out your meals at the start of each week or the night before. Use the supplemental meal planning handout to help you get started. Meal planning must be a priority in your life.

2. Chose several healthy meal options for breakfast, lunch and dinner. This takes the guesswork out of food shopping and meal preparation.

3. Learn the art of "healthy food" label reading. Even "healthy" food marketers can use tricky labeling to draw you to their products. Know what labeling terms actually mean. Review the health labeling terms worksheet on pg. 103-104.

4. Know what to look for when reading a food label. Check the serving size and total calories. Make calories count. Processed foods are high in calories and low in nutrients. Check the sugar content. Check the fat content. Check the sodium content.

KEY CONCEPTS

Chapter 4:
Healthy Eating on the Go

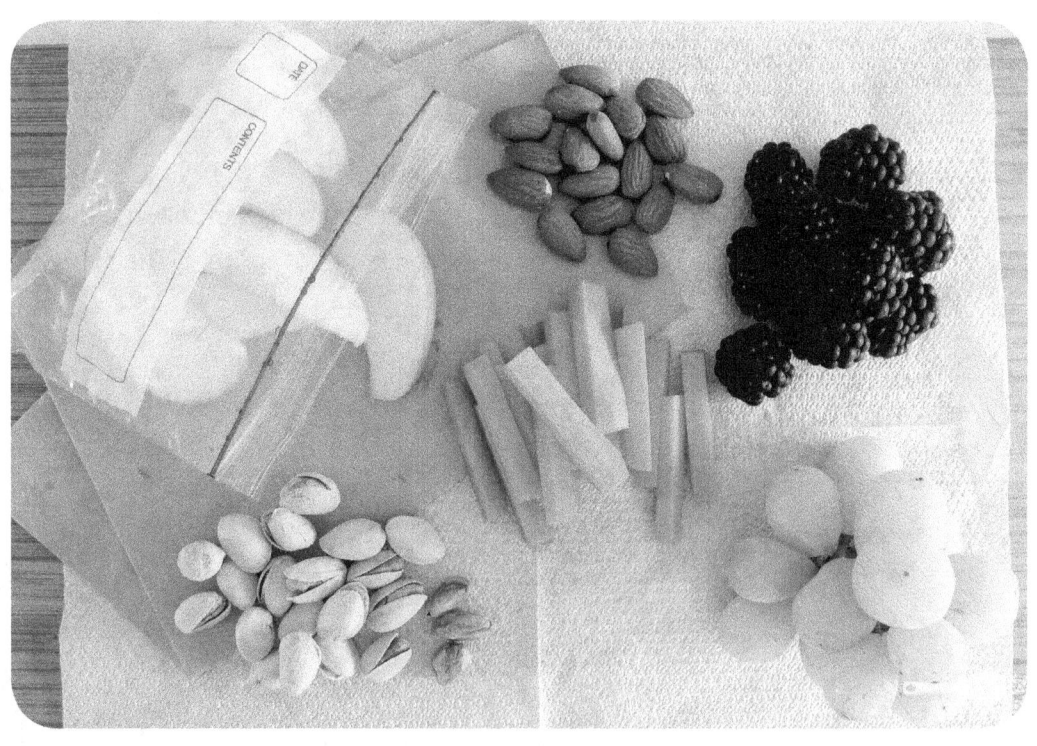

1. When eating out and at restaurants, exercise portion control. You don't have to eat everything on your plate. Save some for another meal or a snack. Request that your food be minimally prepared with low/no added sauces or oils. Avoid eating fried foods. Instead, have your meal steamed, baked, broiled or grilled.

2. When traveling or at social events, plan ahead and bring a healthy alternative or snack to prevent yourself from the temptation of eating unhealthy.

3. Be flexible! Eat your favorite "not-so-healthy-foods" in moderation. Be sure to balance these meals out with nutrient dense meals throughout the same day.

MOVING FORWARD

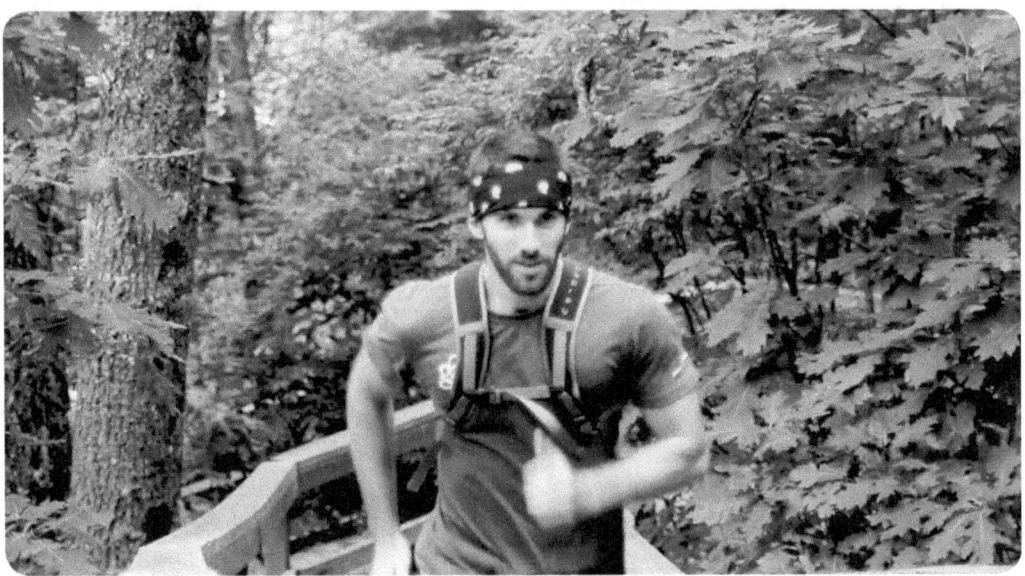

Write down all the changes you've made and are commited to continuing make to eat healthy in the 21st century. These changes may include buying organic food, eating more nutrient dense, plant-based, living foods, incorporating superfoods into your diet, listening to your body and eat according to what it tells you, planning and preparing healthier meals, using the healthy eating on-the-go strategies and techniques, or trying new healthier meal options and recipes.

Changes I am 100% committed to...

1. ....

2. ....

3. ....

4. ....

5. ....

6. ....

7. ....

8. ....

9. ....

10. ....

Congratulations on completing the Healthy Eating in the 21st Century book! By reading this book and following its recommendations, you've taken a massive step toward becoming the healthiest version of you.

I want to encourage you to review all that you have learned and acknowledge and celebrate all the healthy action steps you've already taken and implemented into your life throughout this course. **It is through making small changes now, that lasting results are experienced.**

Now that you've completed this book, it's up to you to put what you've learned into action.

Thanks for taking this journey with me. I truly hope you gain tremendous value from reading it.

Please share your newfound knowledge with your friends and family.

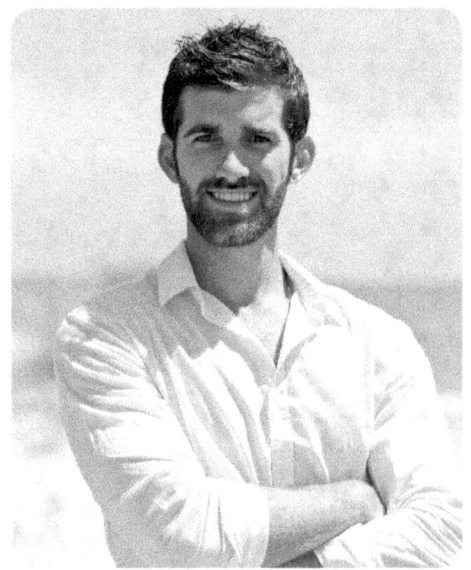

I wish you health, happiness and healthy eating in the 21st century!

Devin Burke
Health and Wellness Coach

For the latest in fitness, wellness and nutrition information follow me!

amazon

Please leave a review.